Copyright © 2021-All rights reserved.

No part of this publication may be reproduced, distributed, or transmitted in any form or by any means, including photocopying, recording, or other electronic or mechanical methods, without the prior written permission of the publisher, except in the case of brief quotations embodied in reviews and certain other non-commercial uses permitted by copyright law.

This Book is provided with the sole purpose of providing relevant information on a specific topic for which every reasonable effort has been made to ensure that it is both accurate and reasonable. Nevertheless, by purchasing this Book you consent to the fact that the author, as well as the publisher, are in no way experts on the topics contained herein, regardless of any claims as such that may be made within. It is recommended that you always consult a professional prior to undertaking any of the advice or techniques discussed with in.This is a legally binding declaration that is considered both valid and fair by both the Committee of Publishers Association and the American Bar Association and should be considered as legally binding within the United States.

CONTENTS

INTRODUCTION **5**
BREAKFAST & BRUNCH **9**
    Zucchini Muffins.. 9
    Chia Pudding with Blackberries............. 9
    Lemon Muffins 10
    Yogurt Strawberry Pie with Basil..........11
STARTERS & SALADS............................... **12**
    Chili Avocado with Cheese Sauce 12
    Chargrilled Broccoli in Tamarind Sauce 13
    Caprese Salad with Bacon......................13
    Tofu Skewers with Sesame Sauce.........14
    Almond Cauliflower Cakes 14
    Roasted Jalapeño & Bell Pepper Soup .15
    Broccoli Salad with Tempeh & Cranberries 15
    Tangy Nutty Brussel Sprout Salad 16
    Pesto Caprese Salad Stacks with Anchovies...16
    Antipasti Skewers.......................................17
    Greek Salad 17
    Buttered Greens with Almonds & Tofu Salad 18
    Zucchini & Dill Bowls with Goat-Feta Cheese 18
    Roasted Bell Pepper Salad with Olives19
    Grandma's Cauliflower Salad with Peanuts 19
    Bruschetta with Tomato & Basil 20
    Speedy Beef Carpaccio 20
    Roasted Asparagus with Goat Cheese..21
    Savory Gruyere & Bacon Cake 21
    Warm Mushroom & Yellow Pepper Salad 22
    Broccoli, Spinach & Feta Salad................22
    Tofu Pops 23
    Blackberry Camembert Puffs 24
    Mini Ricotta Cakes.....................................25
    Mediterranean Roasted Turnip Bites ..26
    Cream Cheese & Caramelized Onion Dip..26
    Tofu Jalapeño Peppers 27
    Avocado Pate with Flaxseed Toasts......27
    Sweet Tahini Twists 28
    Feta Cheese Choux Buns..........................29
SOUPS & STEWS... **30**
    Pork & Pumpkin Stew with Peanuts ... 30
    Paprika Chicken & Bacon Stew............. 30
    Parsley Sausage Stew............................... 31
    Brazilian Moqueca (Shrimp Stew) 31
    Yellow Squash Duck Breast Stew.......... 32
    Herby Chicken Stew 32
LUNCH & DINNER **33**
    Zoodle Bolognese...................................... 33
    Baked Tofu with Roasted Peppers 33
    Spicy Cheese with Tofu Balls 34
    Zucchini Boats with Vegan Cheese...... 34
    Sweet & Spicy Brussel Sprout Stir-Fry 35
    Roasted Butternut Squash with Chimichurri 35
    Tofu Eggplant Pizza 36
    Tomato Artichoke Pizza.......................... 36
    White Pizza with Mixed Mushrooms... 37
    Pepperoni Fat Head Pizza 37
    Vegan Cordon Bleu Casserole............... 38
    Parmesan Meatballs 38
    Seitan Cauliflower Gratin 39
    Walnut Stuffed Mushrooms 39
POULTRY **40**
    Chicken with Tomato and Zucchini 40
    Cauli Rice & Chicken Collard Wraps.... 40
    Almond Crusted Chicken Zucchini Stacks.. 41
    Paleo Coconut Flour Chicken Nuggets 41
    Bacon Chicken Skillet with Bok Choy.. 42
    Celery Chicken Sausage Frittata........... 42
    Rosemary Turkey Brussels Sprouts Cakes 43
    Grilled Garlic Chicken with Cauliflower 43
    Cucumber Salsa Topped Turkey Patties 44
    Turkey with Avocado Sauce................... 44
    Bell Pepper Turkey Keto Carnitas 45
    Caprese Turkey Meatballs 45
    Tasty Curried Chicken Meatballs.......... 46
    Hot Chicken Meatball Tray 46
    Creamy Turkey & Broccoli Bake 47

Cheesy Turkey Sausage Egg Cups 47

BEEF 48
Classic Beef Ragu with Veggie Pasta 48
Barbecued Beef Pizza 48
Beef with Parsnip Noodles 49
Assorted Grilled Veggies & Beef Steaks 49
Classic Swedish Coconut Meatballs 50
Herbed Bolognese Sauce 50
Cheese & Beef Bake 51
Beef Burgers with Roasted Brussels Sprouts 51
Easy Rump Steak Salad 52
Steak Carnitas 52
Tasty Beef Cheeseburgers 53
Beef & Pesto Filled Tomatoes 53
Habanero Beef Cauliflower Pilaf 54
Beef Patties with Cherry Tomatoes 54
Mexican Pizza 55
Beef with Broccoli Rice & Eggs 55
Polish Beef Tripe 56
Smoked Paprika Grilled Ribs 56
Beef Broccoli Curry 57
Shitake Butter Steak 57
Gruyere Beef Burgers with Sweet Onion 58

PORK 59
Pulled Pork Tenderloin with Avocado 59
Broccoli Tips with Lemon Pork Chops 59
Jerk Pork Pot Roast 59
Swiss Pork Patties with Salad 60
Maple Scallion Pork Bites 60
Pork Medallions with Pancetta 61
Golden Pork Chops with Mushrooms .. 61
Cumin Pork Chops 61

SEAFOOD 62
Wine Shrimp Scampi Pizza 62
Shallot Mussel with Shirataki 63
Nori Shrimp Rolls 63
Hazelnut-Crusted Salmon 64
Fish & Cauliflower Parmesan Gratin 64
Broccoli & Fish Gratin 65
Salmon Caesar Salad with Poached Eggs 65
Avocado & Cauliflower Salad with Prawns 66
Fish Fritters 66

VEGAN & VEGETARIAN 67
Mint Ice Cream 67
Eggplant & Goat Cheese Pizza 67
Charred Asparagus with Creamy Sauce 68
Tomato & Mozzarella Caprese Bake 68
Sweet Onion & Goat Cheese Pizza 69
Vegan BBQ Tofu Kabobs with Green Dip 69
One-Pot Spicy Brussel Sprouts with Carrots 70
Tofu Nuggets with Cilantro Dip 70
Zucchini-Cranberry Cake Squares 71
Egg Cauli Fried Rice with Grilled Cheese 71
Strawberry Faux Oats 72
Cheese Quesadillas with Fruit Salad ... 72
Mushroom & Broccoli Pizza 73
Tofu Radish Bowls 73
Mascarpone and Kale Asian Casserole 74
Cauliflower Couscous & Halloumi Packets 74
Mushroom White Pizza 75
Garam Masala Traybake 75
Walnut Chocolate Squares 76
Cauliflower & Broccoli Gratin with Seitan 76
Baked Creamy Brussels Sprouts 77
Mom's Cheesy Pizza 77
Key Lime Truffles 78
Lemon Sponge Cake with Cream 78
Zucchini Cake Slices 79
Blackberry Lemon Tarte Tatin 80
Avocado Truffles with Chocolate Coating 80
Strawberry Blackberry Pie 81
Berry Hazelnut Trifle 81
Coconut Chocolate Fudge 82
Raspberry & Red Wine Crumble 82
Avocado Fries 82
Cacao Nut Bites 83
Cranberry Coconut Parfait 83

SNACKS & SIDE DISHES 84
Jalapeño Nacho Wings 84
Easy Bacon & Cheese Balls 84

Chili Turnip Fries 84
Baked Toast Strips with Prosciutto
Butter 85
Cauliflower Rice & Bacon Gratin 85
Crunchy Rutabaga Puffs 86
Crispy Pancetta & Butternut Squash
Roast 86
Simple Stuffed Eggs with Mayonnaise . 86
Cheesy Pork Rind Bread 87
Savory Lime Fried Artichokes 87
Rosemary Cheese Chips with
Guacamole 87
Parmesan Green Bean Crisps 88
Paprika & Dill Deviled Eggs 88
Cheese & Garlic Crackers 89
Cheesy Chicken Wraps 89
Baked Chorizo with Cottage Cheese 89
Goat Cheese Stuffed Peppers 90
Fried Artichoke Hearts 90
Provolone & Prosciutto Chicken
Wraps 90
Tuna Topped Pickles 91
Keto Deviled Eggs 91
Bacon & Pistachio Liverwurst Truffles 91
Baked Spicy Eggplants 92
Mashed Broccoli with Roasted Garlic .. 92
Spicy Pistachio Dip 93
Prosciutto Appetizer with
Blackberries 93
Onion Rings & Kale Dip 94
Paprika Roasted Nuts 94
Mediterranean Deviled Eggs 95
Mushroom Broccoli Faux Risotto 95
Spinach Chips with Guacamole
Hummus 96
Tofu Stuffed Peppers 96
Soy Chorizo Stuffed Cabbage Rolls 97
Cauliflower Chips with Cheese Dip 97
Mozzarella in Prosciutto Blanket 98
Chocolate, Berries & Nut Mix Bars 98
Chili Avocado-Chimichurri Appetizer . 99
Crispy Squash Nacho Chips 99
Chocolate Walnut Biscuits 100
Herby Cheesy Nuts 100
Mixed Seed Crackers 101
Cheddar and Halloumi Sticks 101
Pesto Mushroom Pinwheels 102
Hemp Seed Zucchini Chips 103
All Seeds Flapjacks 103
Tasty Keto Snickerdoodles 104
Basil-Chili Mozzarella Bites 104

DESSERTS 105
Heart-Shaped Red Velvet Cakes 105
Chocolate Crunch Bars 105
Sticky Maple Cinnamon Cake 106
Almond Square Cookies 106
White Chocolate Chip Cookies 107
Cowboy Cookies 107
Danish Butter Cookies 108
Dark Chocolate Cookies 108
Ginger Cookies 109
Cream Cheese Cookies 109
Easy No-Bake Cookies 110

APPENDIX : RECIPES INDEX 111

INTRODUCTION

Want to follow a ketogenic diet but not sure where to start? Struggling with finding delicious and tummy-filling recipes when going "against the grains"? Do not worry! This book will not only give you amazing keto recipes that will get you started in a jiffy, but it will also teach you the greatest tricks for adopting a keto lifestyle forever.

Mouth-watering delights for any occasion and any eater, you will not believe that these recipes will help you restore your health and slim down your body. Ditching carbs do not mean ditching yummy treats, and with these ingenious recipes, you will see that for yourself.

Successfully practiced for more than nine decades, the ketogenic diet has proven to be the ultimate long-term diet for any person. The restriction list may frighten many, but the truth is, this diet is super adaptable, and the food combinations and tasty meals are pretty endless.

Ketogenic Diet — The New Lifestyle

It is common knowledge that our body is designed to run on carbohydrates. We use them to provide our body with the energy that is required for normal functioning. However, what many people are clueless about, is that carbs are not the only source of fuel that our bodies can use. Just like they can run on carbs, our bodies can also use fats as an energy source. When we ditch the carbs and focus on providing our bodies with more fat, then we are embarking on the ketogenic train.

Despite what many people think, the ketogenic diet is not just another fad diet. It has been around since 1920 and has resulted in outstanding results and amazingly successful stories. If you are new to the keto world and have no idea what I am talking about, let me simplify this for you.

For you to truly understand what the ketogenic diet is all about and why you should choose to follow it, let me first explain what happens to your body after consuming a carb-loaded meal.

Imagine you have just swallowed a giant bowl of spaghetti. Your tummy is full, your taste buds are satisfied, and your body is provided with much more carbs than necessary. After consumption, your body immediately starts the process of digestion, during which your body will break down the consumed carbs into glucose, which is a source of energy that your body depends on. So one might ask," what is wrong with carbs?". There are some things. For starters, they raise the blood sugar, they make us fat, and in short, they hurt our overall health. So, how can ketogenic diet help?

A ketogenic diet skips this process by lowering the carbohydrate intake and providing high fat and moderate protein levels. Now, since there is no adequate amount of carbs to use as energy, your liver is forced to find the fuel elsewhere. And since your body is packed with lots of fat, the liver starts using these extra levels of fat as an energy source.

The Benefits Of The Keto Diet

Despite the fact that it is still considered to be 'controversial,' the keto diet is the best dietary choice that one can make. From weight loss to longevity, here are the benefits that following a ketogenic diet can bring to your life:

<u>Loss of Appetite</u>

Cannot tame your cravings? Do not worry. This diet will neither leave you exhausted nor with a rumbling gut. The ketogenic diet will help you say no to that second piece of cake. Once you train your body to run on fat and not on carbs, you will experience a drop in your appetite that will work magic for your figure.

Weight Loss
Since the body is forced to produce only a small amount of glucose, it will also be forced to lower the insulin production. When that happens, your kidneys will start getting rid of the extra sodium, which will lead to weight loss.

HDL Cholesterol Increase
While consuming a diet high in fat and staying clear of the harmful glucose, your body will experience a rise in the good HDL cholesterol levels, which will, in turn, reduce the risk for many cardiovascular problems.

Drop in Blood Pressure
Cutting back on carbs will also bring your blood pressure in check. The drop in the blood pressure can prevent many health problems such as strokes or heart diseases.

Lower Risk of Diabetes
Although this probably goes without saying, it is important to mention this one. When you ditch the carbs, your body is forced to lower the glucose productivity significantly, which naturally leads to a lower risk of diabetes.

Improved Brain Function
Many studies have shown that replacing carbohydrates with fat as an energy source leads to mental clarity and improved brain function. This is yet another reason why you should go keto.

Longevity
I am not saying that this diet will turn you into a 120-hundred-year-old monk; however, it has been scientifically proven that once the oxidative stress levels are lowered, the lifespan gets extended. And since this diet can result in a significant drop in the oxidative stress levels, the corresponding effect it could have on a person's lifespan is clear.

The Keto Plate

First, just because it is called a 'diet' doesn't mean that you are about to spend your days in starvation. The ketogenic diet will neither tell you not to eat five times a day if you want to nor will it leave your bellies empty.

The only rule that the keto diet has is to eat fewer carbohydrates, more foods that are high in fat, and consume a moderate protein intake. But how much is too much and what is the right amount? The general rule of a thumb is that your daily nutrition should consist of: **70-75% Fat; 20-25% Protein; 5-10% Carbohydrates**

To be more precise, it is not recommended that you consume more than 20 grams of carbs when on a ketogenic diet. This macronutrient percentage, however, can be achieved in whichever way you and your belly are comfortable with. For instance, if you crave a carb meal now, and want to eat, for example, 16 grams of carbs at once, you can do so, as long as your other meals do not contain more than 4 grams of carbs combined.

Some recipes in this book offer 0 grams of carbs, while others are packed with a few grams. By making a proper meal plan that works for you, you can easily skip the inconvenience cloaked around this diet, and start receiving the fantastic benefits.

Keto Flu

The term Keto flu describes a very common experience for new ketoers, but it often goes away in the first week. When starting with keto, you may have some slight discomfort or feel fatigue, headache, nausea, cramps, etc.

The reasons Keto flu occurs are two:

1. Keto diet is diuretic; therefore you visit the bathroom quite often, which leads to the loss of electrolytes and water. The solution is either drinking more water or bouillon cube, to replenish electrolytes reserves. I suggest that you also increase the consumption of potassium, magnesium, calcium, and phosphorus.

2. Shifting to Keto is at first a big shock for the body. The reason is that it's designed to process carbs and now there are almost none. You may feel increased fatigue, nausea, etc. The solution is to decrease carbs intake gradually.

What To Eat
Certain foods will help you up your fat intake and provide you with more longer-lasting energy: Meats, Eggs, Fish and Seafood, Bacon, Sausage, Cacao and sugar-free chocolate, Avocado and berries, Leafy Greens - all of them, Vegetables: cucumber, zucchini, asparagus, broccoli, onion, Brussel sprout, cabbage, tomato, eggplants, seaweed, peppers, squash, Full-Fat Dairy (heavy cream, yogurt, sour cream, cheese, etc.); Nuts — nuts are packed with healthy fats, chestnuts, and cashews, as they contain more carbs than the rest of the nuts. Macadamia nuts, walnuts pecans, and almonds are the best for the Keto diet.; Seeds - chia, flaxseeds, sunflower seeds; Sweeteners - stevia, erythritol, xylitol, monk fruit sugar. I use mostly stevia and erythritol. The latter is a sugar alcohol, but it doesn't spike blood sugar thanks to its zero glycemic indexes; Milk - consume full-fat coconut milk or almond milk; Flour - coconut or almond flour and almond meal; Oils - olive oil, avocado oil; Fats - butter or ghee;

What To Avoid
For you to stay on track with your Keto diet, there are certain foods that you need to say farewell to:
Sugar, honey, agave, soda and sugary drinks, and fruit juices. Starchy vegetables such as potatoes, beans, legumes, peas, yams, and corn are usually packed with tons of carbs, so they must be avoided. However, sneaking some starch when your daily carb limit allows, is not exactly a sin. Flours - all-purpose, wheat, and rice. Dried fruits and fruit in general, except for berries. Grains — rice, wheat, and everything made from grains such as pasta or traditional breads are not allowed. No margarine, milk, refined oils and fats such as corn oil, canola oil, vegetable oil, etc.

Keto Swaps
Just because you are not allowed to eat rice or pasta, doesn't mean that you have to sacrifice eating risotto or spaghetti. Well, sort of. For every forbidden item on the keto diet, there is a healthier replacement that will not contradict your dietary goal and will still taste amazing.
Here are the last keto swaps that you need to know to overcome the cravings quicker, and become a Keto chef:
Bread and Buns Bread made from nut flour, mushroom caps, cucumber slices
Wraps and Tortillas Wraps and tortillas made from nut flour, lettuce leaves, kale leaves
Pasta and Spaghetti Spiralized veggies such as zoodles, spaghetti squash, etc.
Lasagna Noodles Zucchini or eggplant slices
Rice Cauliflower rice (ground in a food processor)
Mashed Potatoes Mashed Cauliflower or other veggies
Hash Browns Cauliflower or Spaghetti squash
Flour Coconut flour, Hazelnut flour, Almond Flour
Breadcrumbs Almond flour

Pizza Crust Crust made with almond flour or cauliflower crust
French Fries Carrot sticks, Turnip fries, Zucchini fries
Potato Chips Zucchini chips, Kale chips
Croutons Bacon bits, nuts, sunflower seeds, flax crackers

Traditional High Carb Comfort Foods Made Keto
Bagel 1 plain 50g net carbs **Low-Carb or FatHead Bagel** 1 plain 4.7g net carbs
Bread 1 slice 12g net carbs **Keto Bread** - 1 slice 1.6g net carbs
Risotto 1 cup 40g net carbs **Cauliflower Risotto** 1 cup 4.2g net carbs
Mashed Potatoes 1 cup 30g net carbs **Mashed Cauliflower** 1 cup 5.3g net carbs
Roasted Potatoes 1 cup 20g net carbs **Roasted Radishes** 1 cup 4.4g net carbs
Pasta 1 cup 40g net carbs **Zoodles/Shirataki Noodles** 1 cup 3.6g/1.3g net carbs
Pepperoni Pizza 1 slice 23g net carbs **Cheesy Bell Pepper Pizza** 3.5g net carbs
Waffle 1 waffle 17g **Keto Waffle** 1 waffle 4.6g net carbs

Getting Started In 5 Easy Steps

1. Time to Revise The Pantry - get rid of all pasta, rice, bread, potatoes, corn, wraps, sugary foods, drinks, legumes, fruits, etc. The less you see those foods, the less you will be tempted to drop on the Keto diet.

2. Get the Basics - now that you've cleaned out your pantry it's time to restock. Your journey toward a healthy and energetic lifestyle has started!

3. Set Up Your Kitchen- cooking delicious food requires additional help from some kitchen appliances. They will make your life easier and the cooking quick and efficient.
My kitchen always has food scales, a blender/food processor, hand mixer, cast iron pans, baking dish, heatproof bowls, and a spiralizer. You will need most of these for the recipes in this cookbook, so I strongly suggest you acquire them to maximize results.

4. Create a Meal Plan - having a meal plan is a great start on the Keto diet. It improves your chances of success, and it's essential for beginners on a diet. That's why my team and I developed a complete 21-Day Meal Plan, which, if followed strictly, would make the transition to Keto diet smooth and delicious.

5. Try to Exercise - your body is designed to be in a constant move. Being on Keto diet isn't going to change that. Yeah, I know that it's difficult and you feel tired. You also have to think constantly about the macros and the food you are eating, but I guarantee you that the more you exercise, the easier you will stick to the diet. Any anaerobic activity would suffice - jogging, running, bicycling, even walking for at least 30 minutes a day will activate your body for optimal performance. I would also suggest some strength exercises but always consult previously on how to train, being on a diet, with your fitness instructor.

BREAKFAST & BRUNCH

Zucchini Muffins

Ingredients for 6 servings
½ cup almond flour
1 tsp baking powder
½ tsp baking soda
1 ½ tsp mustard powder
Salt and black pepper to taste
1/3 cup almond milk
1 large egg
5 tbsp olive oil
½ cup grated cheddar cheese
2 zucchinis, grated
6 green olives, sliced
1 spring onion, chopped
1 red bell pepper, chopped
1 tbsp freshly chopped thyme

Directions and Total Time: approx. 10 minutes
Preheat oven to 325 F. In a bowl, combine flour, baking powder, baking soda, mustard powder, salt, pepper. In a smaller bowl, whisk milk, egg, and olive oil. Mix the wet ingredients into dry ingredients and add cheese, zucchini, olives, spring onion, bell pepper, and thyme; mix well. Spoon the batter into greased muffin cups, and bake for 30 minutes or until golden brown. Let the muffins to cool.
Per serving: Cal 172; Net Carbs 1.6g; Fat 16g; Protein 4g

Chia Pudding with Blackberries

Ingredients for 2 servings
1 cup full-fat natural yogurt
2 tsp swerve
2 tbsp chia seeds
1 cup fresh blackberries
1 tbsp lemon zest
Mint leaves, to serve

Directions and Total Time: approx. 35 minutes
Mix together the yogurt and swerve. Stir in chia seeds. Reserve 4 blackberries for garnish and mash the remaining with a fork until pureed. Stir in the yogurt mixture. Refrigerate for 30 minutes. Divide the mixture into 2 glasses. Serve topped with raspberries and mint leaves.
Per serving: Cal 169, Net Carbs 1.7g, Fat 10g, Protein 7g

Lemon Muffins

Ingredients for 4 servings
For the muffins:
½ cup butter, softened
¾ cup swerve sugar
3 large eggs
1 lemon, zested and juiced
1 ½ cups almond flour
½ cup coconut flour
2 tsp baking powder
¼ tsp arrowroot starch
½ tsp vanilla extract
1 cup sour cream
A pinch of salt
For the topping:
3 tbsp butter, melted
¾ cup almond flour
3 Tbsp swerve sugar
1 tsp lemon zest
1 tbsp coconut flour
For the lemon glaze:
½ cup swerve confectioner's sugar
3 tbsp lemon juice

Directions and Total Time: approx. 35 minutes
For the muffins:
Preheat oven to 350 F and line a 12-cup muffin pan with paper liners. In a bowl, mix butter, swerve, eggs, lemon zest, and lemon juice until smooth. In another bowl, combine flours, baking powder, and arrowroot. Combine both mixtures and mix in vanilla, sour cream, and salt until smooth. Fill the cups two-thirds way up; set aside.
For the topping:
In a bowl, mix butter, almond flour, swerve, lemon zest, and coconut flour until well combined. Spoon the mixture onto the muffin batter and bake for 25 minutes or until a toothpick inserted comes out clean. Remove the muffins from the oven and cool while you prepare the glaze.
For the glaze:
In a bowl, whisk confectioner's sugar and lemon juice until smooth and semi-thick. Drizzle over the muffins.
Per serving: Cal 439; Net Carbs 7.6g; Fat 42g; Protein 8g

Yogurt Strawberry Pie with Basil

Ingredients for 4 servings

For the crust:
2 eggs
1 tsp vanilla extract
¼ cup erythritol
¼ tsp salt
1 cup almond flour
½ cup cold butter, cubed
5 tbsp cold water
1 tbsp olive oil

For the filling:
1 cup unsweetened strawberry jam
¼ cup heavy cream
1/3 cup erythritol
1 cup Greek yogurt
1 tbsp chopped basil leaves

Directions and Total Time: approx. 90 min + chilling time

For the piecrust:
In a bowl, whisk eggs, olive oil, and vanilla until well combined. In another bowl, mix erythritol, salt, and flour. Combine both mixtures into a stand mixer and blend until smooth dough forms. Add butter and mix until breadcrumb-like mixture forms. Add one tbsp of water, mix further until the dough begins to come together. Keep adding water until it sticks together. Lightly flour a working surface, turn the dough onto it, knead a few times until formed into a ball, and comes together smoothly. Divide into half and flatten each piece into a disk. Wrap each dough in plastic and refrigerate for 1 hour. Preheat oven to 375 F and grease a 9-inch pie pan with olive oil. Remove the dough from the fridge, let it stand at room temperature and roll one piece into 12-inch round. Fit this piece into the bottom and walls to the rim of the pie pan while shaping to take the pan's form. Roll out the other dough into an 11-inch round and set aside.

For the filling:
Whip the heavy cream and erythritol in a stand mixer until creamy and smooth. Mix in the Greek yogurt, strawberry jam, basil and mix on low speed until well combined. Fill the pie dough in the pie pan with the filling and level well. Brush the overhanging pastry with water and attach the top pastry on top of the filling. Press the edges to merge the dough ends and trim the overhanging ends to 1-inch. Fold the edge under itself and then, decoratively crimp. Cut 2 slits on the top crust. Bake the pie for 75 minutes until the bottom crust is golden and the filling bubbly.

Per serving: Cal 341; Net Carbs 6.1g; Fat 33g; Protein 5.6g

STARTERS & SALADS

Chili Avocado with Cheese Sauce

Ingredients for 4 servings
5 tbsp melted butter
3 tbsp almond flour
1 ½ cups almond milk
¼ tsp mustard powder
¼ tsp garlic powder
Black pepper to taste
1 cup grated cheddar cheese
4 oz cream cheese, softened
¼ cup grated Parmesan
2 avocados, sliced
2 tbsp sriracha sauce
2 tbsp olive oil

Directions and Total Time: approx. 16 minutes
Mix 3 tbsps of butter with flour in a saucepan and cook until golden. Whisk in milk, mustard, garlic, and black pepper. Cook, whisking continuously until thickened, 2 minutes. Stir in cheddar, cream and Parmesan cheeses until melted; set aside. In a bowl, toss avocado in remaining butter and sriracha sauce. Heat olive oil in a pan and cook avocado until golden turning halfway, 4 minutes. Plate and pour the cheese sauce all over to serve.
Per serving: Cal 548; Net Carbs 3.2g; Fat 49g; Protein 10g

Chargrilled Broccoli in Tamarind Sauce

Ingredients for 6 servings
1 head broccoli, cut into florets
4 tbsp melted butter
1 white onion, finely chopped
3 garlic cloves, minced
1 tsp dried basil
Salt and black pepper to taste
A handful of chopped parsley
1 garlic clove, peeled
1 inch ginger, peeled
½ lemon, juiced
½ cup peanut butter
2 tbsp tamarind sauce
1 tsp swerve brown sugar
1 small red chili, chopped

Directions and Total Time: approx. 30 minutes
Simmer 2 cups of water in a pot and blanch broccoli for 2 minutes; drain. In a bowl, mix butter, onion, garlic, basil, salt, pepper. Toss broccoli in the mixture and marinate for 5 minutes. Heat a grill pan over high and cook broccoli until charred, turning once. Transfer to a plate. Place garlic and ginger in a blender and pulse until broken into pieces. Add in lemon juice, peanut butter, tamarind sauce, brown sugar, red chili, and 1/3 cup of water. Blend until smooth. Serve broccoli topped with peanut sauce and parsley.

Per serving: Cal 269; Net Carbs 5.2g; Fat 18g; Protein 7.6g

Caprese Salad with Bacon

Ingredients for 2 servings
1 tomato, sliced
4 basil leaves
8 mozzarella cheese slices
2 tsp olive oil
3 ounces bacon, chopped
1 tsp balsamic vinegar

Directions and Total Time: approx. 10 minutes
Place the bacon in a skillet over medium heat and cook until crispy. Divide the tomato slices between 2 serving plates. Arrange the mozzarella slices on top.
Scatter basil leaves and add the bacon on top. Drizzle with olive oil and vinegar. Sprinkle with sea salt and serve.

Per serving: Cal 279; Net Carbs 1.5g; Fat 26g; Protein 21g

Tofu Skewers with Sesame Sauce

Ingredients for 4 servings
2 tbsp tahini
1 (14 oz) firm tofu, cubed
1 zucchini, cut into wedges
¼ cup cherry tomatoes, halved
1 red onion, cut into wedges
1 tbsp soy sauce
1 tbsp olive oil
Sesame seeds for garnishing

Directions and Total Time: approx. 15 minutes
In a bowl, mix tahini and soy sauce; mix toss tofu in the sauce. Let rest for 30 minutes. Thread tofu, zucchini, tomatoes and onion, alternately, on wooden skewers. Heat olive oil in a grill pan and cook tofu until golden brown, 8 minutes. Serve garnished with sesame seeds.
Per serving: Cal 266; Net Carbs 2.4g; Fat 19g; Protein 14g

Almond Cauliflower Cakes

Ingredients for 4 servings
½ cup grated Parmigiano Reggiano cheese
2 cups cauliflower florets
Salt and black pepper to taste
1 large egg, beaten
2 green onions, chopped
1 tbsp chopped parsley
2 tbsp chopped almonds
1 cup golden flaxseed meal
1 cup olive oil

Directions and Total Time: approx. 25 minutes
Pour cauliflower and 1 cup of water into a pot and bring to a boil until soft; drain. Transfer to a food processor and puree until smooth. Pour into a bowl and mix in salt, pepper, egg, green onions, parsley, cheese, and almonds. Make 12 small cakes from the mixture and coat in the flaxseed meal. Heat olive oil a deep pan and cook patties on both sides until golden, 6-8 minutes. Serve warm.
Per serving: Cal 321; Net Carbs 5.5g; Fat 23g; Protein 14g

Roasted Jalapeño & Bell Pepper Soup

Ingredients for 4 servings
6 green bell peppers, halved
1 jalapeño pepper, halved
1 bulb garlic, halved, not peeled
6 tomatoes, halved
3 cups vegetable broth
2 tbsp melted butter
½ cup heavy cream
3 tbsp grated Parmesan
Roughly chopped chives
Salt and black pepper to taste

Directions and Total Time: approx. 40 minutes
Preheat oven to 350 F. Arrange bell peppers, jalapeño pepper, and garlic on a baking pan and roast for 15 minutes. Add tomatoes roast for 15 minutes. Let cool, peel of the skins, and place in a blender. Add salt, pepper, butter, and heavy cream; puree until completely smooth. Serve into bowls, sprinkle with Parmesan and chives.
Per serving: Cal 189; Net Carbs 8.7g; Fat 12g; Protein 5.3g

Broccoli Salad with Tempeh & Cranberries

Ingredients for 4 servings
3 oz vegan butter
¾ lb tempeh slices, cubed
1 lb broccoli florets
Salt and black pepper to taste
2 oz almonds
½ cup frozen cranberries

Directions and Total Time: approx. 10 minutes
In a deep skillet, melt vegan butter over medium heat and fry tempeh cubes until brown on all sides. Add in broccoli and stir-fry for 6 minutes. Season with salt and pepper. Turn the heat off. Stir in almonds and cranberries to warm through. Share the salad into bowls and serve.
Per serving: Cal 740; Net Carbs 7g; Fat 72g; Protein 12g

Tangy Nutty Brussel Sprout Salad

Ingredients for 4 servings
1 lb Brussels sprouts, grated
1 lemon, juice and zest
½ cup olive oil
Salt and black pepper to taste
1 tbsp vegan butter
1 tsp chili paste
2 oz pecans
1 oz pumpkin seeds
1 oz sunflower seeds
½ tsp cumin powder

Directions and Total Time: approx. 20 minutes
Place Brussels sprouts in a salad bowl. In a bowl, mix lemon juice, zest, olive oil, salt, and pepper, and drizzle the dressing over Brussels sprouts. Toss and let marinate for 10 minutes. Melt vegan butter in a pan. Stir in chili paste, pecans, pumpkin and sunflower seeds, cumin powder, and salt. Cook on low heat for 4 minutes just to heat up; let cool. Mix nuts and seeds with Brussel sprouts to serve.
Per serving: Cal 420; Net Carbs 8g; Fat 35g; Protein 12g

Pesto Caprese Salad Stacks with Anchovies

Ingredients for 4 servings
4 red tomato slices
4 yellow tomato slices
12 fresh mozzarella slices
1 cup basil pesto
4 anchovy fillets in oil

Directions and Total Time: approx. 10 minutes
On a serving platter, alternately stack a tomato slice, a mozzarella slice, an yellow tomato slice, another mozzarella slice, a red tomato slice, and then one a mozzarella slice. Repeat making 3 more stacks in the same way. Spoon pesto all over. Arrange anchovies on top to serve.
Per serving: Cal 178; Net Carbs 3.5g; Fat 6.1g; Protein 17g

Antipasti Skewers

Ingredients for 4 servings
4 zucchini lengthwise slices
8 cubes cheddar cheese
4 mini bamboo skewers
8 cherry tomatoes
8 fresh mint leaves

Directions and Total Time: approx. 45 minutes
Lay zucchini slices on a flat surface and place 2 cheddar cubes on one end of each slice. Wrap zucchini around the cheese cubes and insert a skewer each to secure. Alternately, thread the tomatoes and mint leaves onto the skewers and season with salt. Place the skewers on a plate, cover with plastic wrap, and chill for 30 minutes. Serve.
Per serving: Cal 93; Net Carbs 1.8g; Fat 3.9g; Protein 7g

Greek Salad

Ingredients for 2 servings
½ yellow bell pepper, sliced
3 tomatoes, sliced
½ cucumber, sliced
½ red onion, sliced thinly
½ cup tofu cheese, cubed
10 Kalamata olives, pitted
½ tbsp red wine vinegar
4 tbsp olive oil
Salt and ground black pepper
2 tsp dried oregano

Directions and Total Time: approx. 10 minutes
Pour bell pepper, tomatoes, cucumber, red onion, and tofu cheese in a bowl. Drizzle red wine vinegar and olive oil all over and season with salt, pepper, and oregano; toss to coat. Transfer to a salad platter, top with olives, and serve.
Per serving: Cal 580; Net Carbs 13g; Fat 49g; Protein 15g

Buttered Greens with Almonds & Tofu Salad

Ingredients for 4 servings
2 tbsp olive oil
1 (7 oz) block tofu, cubed
2 tbsp butter
1 cup green beans, trimmed
1 cup asparagus, halved
Salt and black pepper to taste
½ lemon, juiced
4 tbsp chopped almonds

Directions and Total Time: approx. 25 minutes
Heat olive oil in a skillet and fry the tofu until golden, 10 minutes; set aside. Add butter to the skillet and pour in green beans and asparagus; season with salt and pepper, toss and cook until softened. Mix in tofu and stir-fry further for 5 minutes. Drizzle with lemon juice and scatter almonds on top. Serve warm.

Per serving: Cal 237; Net Carbs 3.9g; Fat 15g; Protein 13g

Zucchini & Dill Bowls with Goat-Feta Cheese

Ingredients for 4 servings
4 zucchinis, spiralized
Salt and black pepper to taste
½ lemon, zested and juiced
1 tbsp olive oil
¼ tsp Dijon mustard
1 tbsp chopped dill leaves
½ cup baby kale
1/3 cup crumbled goat cheese
1/3 cup crumbled feta cheese
2 tbsp toasted pine nuts

Directions and Total Time: approx. 35 minutes
Put the zucchinis in a bowl and season with salt and pepper. In a small bowl, mix the lemon juice, olive oil, and mustard. Pour the mixture over the zucchini and toss evenly. Add the dill, kale, goat cheese, feta cheese, and pine nuts. Toss to combine and serve.

Per serving: Cal 457; Net Carbs 9.5g; Fat 36g; Protein 26g

Roasted Bell Pepper Salad with Olives

Ingredients for 4 servings
8 large red bell peppers, deseeded and cut in wedges
½ tsp swerve sugar
2 ½ tbsp olive oil
1/3 cup arugula
1/3 cup pitted Kalamata olives
1 tbsp mint leaves
3 tbsp toasted chopped walnuts
½ tbsp balsamic vinegar
Crumbled goat cheese
Toasted pine nuts for topping
Salt and black pepper to taste

Directions and Total Time: approx. 30 minutes
Preheat oven to 400 F. Pour bell peppers on a roasting pan; season with swerve sugar and drizzle with half of the olive oil. Roast for 20 minutes or until slightly charred; set aside to cool. Put arugula in a salad bowl and scatter with roasted bell peppers, olives, mint, walnuts, and drizzle with vinegar and olive oil. Season with salt and pepper. Toss, top with goat cheese and pine nuts and serve.
Per serving: Cal 163; Net Carbs 4.3g; Fat 13g; Protein 3.3g

Grandma's Cauliflower Salad with Peanuts

Ingredients for 4 servings
1 small head cauliflower, cut into florets
12 green olives, chopped
8 sun-dried tomatoes, drained
3 tbsp chopped scallions
1 lemon, zested and juiced
2 tbsp sesame oil
A handful of toasted peanuts
3 tbsp chopped parsley
½ cup watercress
Salt and black pepper to taste
Lemon wedges to garnish

Directions and Total Time: approx. 20 minutes
Bring water to a boil in a pot. Pour cauliflower into a steamer basket and soften over the boiling water, 10 minutes. Transfer cauliflower to a salad bowl. Add in olives, tomatoes, scallions, lemon zest and juice, sesame oil, peanuts, parsley, and watercress. Season with salt, pepper, and mix using a spoon. Serve with lemon wedges.
Per serving: Cal 203; Net Carbs 6.4g; Fat 15g; Protein 6.6g

Bruschetta with Tomato & Basil

Ingredients for 4 servings
3 ripe tomatoes, chopped
6 fresh basil leaves
5 tbsp olive oil
Salt to taste
4 slices zero carb bread, halved
1 garlic clove, halved

Directions and Total Time: approx. 1 hour 15 minutes
In a bowl, mix tomatoes and basil until combined. Drizzle with 2 tbsp olive oil and salt; do not stir. Set aside.
Brush bread slices with the remaining olive oil, arrange on a baking sheet, and place under the broiler. Cook for 2 minutes per side or until lightly browned. Transfer to a plate and rub garlic on both sides. Cover with tomato topping. Drizzle a little more of olive oil on top and serve.
Per serving: Cal 212; Net Carbs 2.7g; Fat 19g; Protein 8g

Speedy Beef Carpaccio

Ingredients for 4 servings
1 tbsp olive oil
½ lemon, juiced
Salt and black pepper to taste
¼ lb rare roast beef, sliced
1 ½ cups baby arugula
¼ cup grated Parmesan cheese

Directions and Total Time: approx. 10 minutes
In a bowl, whisk olive oil, lemon juice, salt, and pepper until well combined. Spread the beef on a large serving plate, top with arugula and drizzle the olive oil mixture on top. Sprinkle with grated Parmesan cheese and serve.
Per serving: Cal 106; Net Carbs 4.1g; Fat 5g; Protein 10g

Roasted Asparagus with Goat Cheese

Ingredients for 4 servings
1 lb asparagus, halved
2 tbsp olive oil
½ tsp dried tarragon
½ tsp dried oregano
½ tsp sesame seeds
1 tbsp sugar-free maple syrup
½ cup arugula
4 tbsp crumbled goat cheese
2 tbsp hazelnuts
1 lemon, cut into wedges

Directions and Total Time: approx. 30 minutes
Preheat oven to 350 F. Pour asparagus on a baking tray, drizzle with olive oil, tarragon, oregano, salt, pepper, and sesame seeds. Toss and roast for 15 minutes; remove and drizzle the maple syrup, and continue cooking for 5 minutes or until slightly charred. Spread arugula in a salad bowl and spoon the asparagus on top. Scatter with the goat cheese, hazelnuts, and serve with the lemon wedges.
Per serving: Cal 146; Net Carbs 3.4g; Fat 13g; Protein 4.4g

Savory Gruyere & Bacon Cake

Ingredients for 4 servings
½ cup shredded Gruyere cheese
4 eggs, eggs yolks and whites separated
2 tbsp butter
2 tbsp almond flour
1 cup heavy cream
6 slices bacon, chopped

Directions and Total Time: approx. 50 minutes
Melt butter in a pan over medium heat and mix in 1 tbsp of almond flour until well combined. Whisk in heavy cream, bring to a boil and while stirring, mix in the remaining almond flour until smooth. Turn the heat off. Cool the mixture for 3 minutes and slowly mix the batter into the egg yolks until well combined without cooking. Stir in Gruyere cheese until evenly distributed. Beat the egg whites in a mixer until stiff peak forms.
Fold the egg whites into the egg yolk mixture until well combined. Divide the mixture between 4 ramekins, top with bacon and bake in the oven for 35 minutes at 320 F.
Per serving: Cal 495; Net Carbs 2g, Fat 46g, Protein 17.3g

Warm Mushroom & Yellow Pepper Salad

Ingredients for 4 servings
1 cup mixed mushrooms, chopped
2 tbsp sesame oil
2 yellow bell peppers, sliced
1 garlic clove, minced
2 tbsp tamarind sauce
½ tsp hot sauce
1 tsp sugar-free maple syrup
½ tsp ginger paste
Salt and black pepper to taste
Chopped toasted pecans
Sesame seeds to garnish

Directions and Total Time: approx. 20 minutes
Heat half of the sesame oil in a skillet, sauté bell peppers and mushrooms for 8-10 minutes; season with salt and pepper. In a bowl, mix garlic, tamarind sauce, hot sauce, maple syrup, and ginger paste. Stir the mix into the vegetables and stir-fry for 2-3 minutes. Divide salad between 4 plates; drizzle with the remaining sesame oil and garnish with pecans and sesame seeds. Serve.
Per serving: Cal 289; Net Carbs 5.2g; Fat 27g; Protein 4.2g

Broccoli, Spinach & Feta Salad

Ingredients for 4 servings
2 tbsp olive oil
1 tbsp white wine vinegar
2 tbsp poppy seeds
Salt and black pepper to taste
2 cups broccoli slaw
2 cups chopped spinach
1/3 cup chopped walnuts
1/3 cup sunflower seeds
1/3 cup blueberries
2/3 cup chopped feta cheese

Directions and Total Time: approx. 15 minutes
In a bowl, whisk olive oil, vinegar, poppy seeds, salt, and pepper; set aside. In a salad bowl, combine the broccoli slaw, spinach, walnuts, sunflower seeds, blueberries, and feta cheese. Drizzle the dressing on top, toss, and serve.
Per serving: Cal 397; Net Carbs 4.9g; Fat 3.8g; Protein 9g

Tofu Pops

Ingredients for 4 servings
1 (14 oz) block tofu, cubed
1 bunch of chives, chopped
1 lemon, zested and juiced
12 slices bacon
12 mini skewers
1 tsp butter

Directions and Total Time: approx. 1 hour 17 minutes
Mix chives, lemon zest, and juice in a bowl and toss the tofu cubes in the mixture. Marinate for 1 hour. Remove the zest and chives off the cubes and wrap each tofu in a bacon slice; insert each skewer and the end of the bacon. Melt butter in a skillet and fry tofu skewers until the bacon browns and crisps. Serve with mayo dipping sauce.
Per serving: Cal 392; Net Carbs 9g, Fat 22g, Protein 18g

Blackberry Camembert Puffs

Ingredients for 4 servings
For the pastry cups:
¼ cup butter, cold and crumbled
¼ cup almond flour
3 tbsp coconut flour
½ tsp xanthan gum
½ tsp salt
4 tbsp cream cheese, softened
1/4 teaspoon cream of tartar
3 whole eggs, unbeaten
3 tbsp erythritol
1 ½ tsp vanilla extract
1 whole egg, beaten

For the filling:
5 oz Camembert, sliced and cut into 16 cubes
1 tsp butter
1 yellow onion, chopped
3 tbsp red wine
1 tbsp balsamic vinegar
5 tbsp erythritol
½ cup fresh blackberries
Freshly parsley to garnish

Directions and Total Time: approx. 30 minutes
Preheat oven to 350 F, turn a muffin tray upside down and lightly grease with cooking spray. In a bowl, mix almond and coconut flours, xanthan gum, and salt. Add in cream cheese, cream of tartar, and butter; mix with an electric hand mixer until crumbly. Stir in erythritol and vanilla extract until mixed. Then, pour in three eggs, one after another while mixing until formed into a ball. Flatten the dough on a clean flat surface, cover in plastic wrap, and refrigerate for 1 hour. Dust a clean flat surface with almond flour, unwrap the dough, and roll out the dough into a large rectangle. Cut into 16 squares and press each onto each muffin mound on the tray to form a bowl shape. Brush with the remaining eggs and bake for 10 minutes.

To make the filling, melt butter in a skillet and sauté onion for 3 minutes. Stir in red wine, balsamic vinegar, erythritol, and blackberries. Cook until the berries become jammy and wine reduces, 10 minutes. Set aside. Take out the tray and place a cheese cubes in each pastry. Return to oven and bake for 3 minutes. Spoon a tsp each of the blackberry sauce on top. Garnish with parsley to serve.

Per serving: Cal 372; Net Carbs 4.4g, Fat 32g, Protein 14g

Mini Ricotta Cakes

Ingredients for 4 servings
2 tbsp olive oil
2 tbsp butter
2 garlic cloves, minced
1 white onion, finely chopped
1 cup cauli rice
¼ cup white wine
¼ cup vegetable stock
2 scallions, chopped
Salt and black pepper to taste
¼ cup grated Parmesan
½ cup ricotta cheese
1 cup almond flour
½ cup golden flaxseed meal
2 eggs

Directions and Total Time: approx. 40 minutes
Heat butter in a saucepan over medium heat. Stir in garlic and onion and cook until fragrant and soft, 3 minutes. Mix in cauli rice for 30 seconds; add in wine, stir, allow reduction and absorption into cauli rice.

Mix in stock, scallions, salt, pepper, remaining butter, Parmesan and ricotta cheeses. Cover the pot and cook until the liquid reduces and the rice thickens. Open the lid, stir well, and spoon the mixture into a bowl to cool. Mold the dough into mini patties, about 14 to 16 and set aside. Heat olive oil in a skillet over medium heat; meanwhile pour the almond flour onto a plate, the golden flaxseed meal in another, and beat the eggs in a medium bowl. Lightly dredge each patty in the flour, then in eggs, and then coated accurately in the flaxseed meal. Fry in the oil until compacted and golden brown, 2 minutes on each side. Transfer to a paper towel-lined plate, plate, and garnish with some scallions.

Per serving: Cal 362; Net Carbs 6.2g, Fat 29g, Protein 13g

Mediterranean Roasted Turnip Bites

Ingredients for 4 servings
1 lb turnips, sliced into rounds
½ cup olive oil
2 garlic cloves, minced
1 tbsp chopped fresh parsley
2 tbsp chopped fresh oregano
3 tbsp dried Italian seasoning
¼ cup marinara sauce
¼ cup grated mozzarella

Directions and Total Time: approx. 1 hour
Preheat oven to 400 F. Place turnip slices into a bowl and toss with olive oil. Add in garlic, parsley, oregano, and Italian seasoning and mix well. Arrange on a greased baking sheet and roast for 25 minutes, flipping halfway. Remove and brush the marinara sauce. Sprinkle with mozzarella cheese and bake in the oven until the cheese is golden, 15 minutes. Garnish with parsley and serve warm.
Per serving: Cal 326; Net Carbs 3.8g; Fat 28g; Protein 5g

Cream Cheese & Caramelized Onion Dip

Ingredients for 4 servings
2 tbsp butter
3 yellow onions, thinly sliced
1 tsp swerve sugar
Salt to taste
¼ cup white wine
2 cups sour cream
8 oz cream cheese, softened
½ tbsp Worcestershire sauce

Directions and Total Time: approx. 30 minutes
Melt butter in a skillet and add in onions, swerve sugar, and salt and cook with frequent stirring for 10-15 minutes. Add in white wine, stir and allow sizzling out, 10 minutes. In a serving bowl, mix sour cream and cream cheese until well combined. Add onions and Worcestershire sauce; stir well into the cream. Serve with celery sticks.
Per serving: Cal 383; Net Carbs 8.3g; Fat 34g; Protein 8g

Tofu Jalapeño Peppers

Ingredients for 4 servings
For the poppers:
1 tbsp olive oil
4 oz firm tofu, chopped in bits
1 garlic clove, minced
½ cup cream cheese
1 lemon, zested juiced
4 scallions, finely chopped
2 tbsp chopped cilantro
Salt and black pepper to taste
6 jalapeño peppers, halved
3 tbsp grated cheddar cheese
For the dip:
1 tsp lemon juice
1 cup sour cream
1 tbsp chopped cilantro

Directions and Total Time: approx. 30 minutes
Preheat oven to 370 F. Heat olive oil in a skillet and fry tofu until golden. Transfer to a bowl. Mix in garlic, cream cheese, lemon zest, juice, scallions, cilantro, salt, and pepper. Arrange jalapeño peppers on a greased baking dish. Fill tofu mixture and sprinkle with cheddar cheese. Bake for 15 minutes or until the cheese is golden brown. In a bowl, mix lemon juice, sour cream, cilantro, and season with salt and pepper. Serve the dip with the poppers.
Per serving: Cal 247; Net Carbs 6.9g, Fat 21g, Protein 9g

Avocado Pate with Flaxseed Toasts

Ingredients for 4 servings
1/2 cup flaxseed meal
1 pinch salt
For the Avocado pate:
3 ripe avocado, chopped
4 tbsp Greek yogurt
2 tbsp chopped green onions
1 lemon, zested and juiced
Black pepper to taste
Smoked paprika to garnish

Directions and Total Time: approx. 5 minutes
For the flaxseed toasts:
Preheat oven to 350 F. Place a skillet over medium heat. Mix in flaxseed meal, 1/4 cup water, and salt and mix continually to form the dough into a ball. Place the dough between 2 parchment papers, put on a flat surface, and flatten thinly with a rolling pin. Remove the papers and cut the pastry into tortilla chips. Place on a baking sheet and bake for 8-12 minutes or until crispy. In a bowl, mix avocado, yogurt, green onions, lemon zest, juice, and black pepper until evenly combined. Spread the pate on the toasts and garnish with paprika. Serve immediately.
Per serving: Cal 364; Net Carbs 4g, Fat 31g, Protein 7.4g

Sweet Tahini Twists

Ingredients for 4 servings
For the puff pastry:
¼ cup almond flour
3 tbsp coconut flour
½ tsp xanthan gum
½ tsp salt
4 tbsp cream cheese, softened
¼ teaspoon cream of tartar
¼ cup butter, cold
3 whole eggs
3 tbsp erythritol
1 ½ tsp vanilla extract
1 whole egg, beaten
For the filling:
2 tbsp sugar-free maple syrup
3 tbsp tahini
2 tbsp sesame seeds
1 egg, beaten
2 tbsp poppy seeds

Directions and Total Time: approx. 15 min + cooling time
Preheat oven to 350 F and line a baking tray with parchment paper. In a bowl, mix almond and coconut flours, xanthan gum, and salt. Add in cream cheese, cream of tartar, and butter; mix with an electric mixer until crumbly. Add erythritol and vanilla extract until mixed. Then, pour in 3 eggs one after another while mixing until formed into a ball. Flatten the dough on a clean flat surface, cover in plastic wrap, and refrigerate for 1 hour.
Dust a clean flat surface with almond flour, unwrap the dough, and roll out the dough into a large rectangle. In a bowl, mix sugar-free maple syrup with tahini and spread the mixture over the pastry. Sprinkle with half of the sesame seeds and cut the dough into 16 thin strips. Fold each strip in half. Brush the top with the remaining egg, sprinkle with the remaining seeds, and poppy seeds. Twist the pastry three to four times into straws and place on the baking sheet. Bake until golden brown, 15 minutes. Serve with chocolate sauce.
Per serving: Cal 348; Net Carbs 3.1g, Fat 31g, Protein 11g

Feta Cheese Choux Buns

Ingredients for 4 servings

2 sprigs rosemary
6 tbsp butter
2/3 cup almond flour
3 eggs, beaten
1 tbsp olive oil
2 white onions, thinly sliced
2 tbsp red wine vinegar
1 tsp swerve brown sugar
1 cup crumbled feta cheese
½ cup heavy whipping cream

Directions and Total Time: approx. 40 minutes

Preheat oven to 350 F and line a baking tray with parchment paper. In a saucepan, warm 1 cup of water, salt, and butter melts. Bring to a boil and sift in flour, beating vigorously until ball forms. Turn the heat off; keep beating while adding the eggs, one at a time, until the dough is smooth and slightly thickened. Scoop mounds of the dough onto the baking dish. Press a hole in the center of each mound. Bake for 20 minutes until risen and golden. Remove from oven and pierce the sides of the buns with a toothpick. Return to oven and bake for 2 minutes until crispy. Set aside to cool.

Tear out the middle part of the bun (keep the torn out part) to create a hole in the bun for the cream filling. Set aside. Heat olive oil in a saucepan and sauté onions and rosemary for 2 minutes. Stir in swerve, vinegar, and cook to bubble for 3 minutes or until caramelized. In a bowl, beat whipping cream and feta together. Spoon the mixture into a piping bag and press a spoonful of the mixture into the buns. Cover with the torn out portion of pastry and top with onion relish to serve.

Per serving: Cal 384; Net Carbs 2.5g, Fat 37g, Protein 10g

SOUPS & STEWS

Pork & Pumpkin Stew with Peanuts

Ingredients for 6 servings
1 cup puree
2 lb pork shoulder, cubed
1 tbsp peanut butter
4 tbsp chopped peanuts
1 garlic clove, minced
½ cup chopped onion
½ cup white wine
1 tbsp olive oil
1 tsp lemon juice
¼ cup granulated sweetener
¼ tsp cardamom
¼ tsp allspice
3 cups chicken stock
Salt and black pepper to taste

Directions and Total Time: approx. 45 minutes
Heat olive oil in a pot. Add onions and garlic and sauté for 3 minutes. Add in pork and stir-fry for 5-6 minutes. Pour in wine and cook for 1 minute. Throw in the remaining ingredients, except lemon juice and peanuts. Bring the mixture to a boil, and cook for 5 minutes. Reduce the heat and let cook for 30 minutes. Adjust seasoning. Stir in lemon juice before serving. Serve topped with peanuts.
Per serving: Cal 451; Net Carbs 4g; Fat 33g, Protein 27.5g

Paprika Chicken & Bacon Stew

Ingredients for 3 servings
8 bacon strips, chopped
¼ cup Dijon mustard
Salt and black pepper to taste
1 onion, chopped
1 tbsp olive oil
1 ½ cups chicken stock
3 chicken breasts
¼ tsp sweet paprika

Directions and Total Time: approx. 40 minutes
In a bowl, combine salt, pepper, and mustard. Massage onto chicken breasts. Set a pan over medium heat, stir in the bacon, cook until it browns, and remove to a plate. Heat oil in the same pan, add the breasts, cook each side for 2 minutes, set aside. Place in the stock and bring to a simmer. Stir in pancetta and onions. Return the chicken to the pan as well, stir gently, and simmer for 20 minutes over medium heat, turning halfway through. Serve.
Per serving: Cal 313; Net Carbs 3g; Fat 18g, Protein 26g

Parsley Sausage Stew

Ingredients for 6 servings
1 lb pork sausage, sliced
1 red bell pepper, chopped
1 onion, chopped
Salt and black pepper, to taste
1 cup fresh parsley, chopped
6 green onions, chopped
¼ cup avocado oil
1 cup chicken stock
2 garlic cloves, minced
24 ounces canned tomatoes
16 ounces okra, sliced
6 ounces tomato sauce
2 tbsp coconut aminos
1 tbsp hot sauce

Directions and Total Time: approx. 35 minutes
Set a pot over medium heat and warm oil. Place in sausages and cook for 2 minutes. Stir in onion, green onions, garlic, black pepper, bell pepper, and salt, and cook for 5 minutes. Add in hot sauce, stock, tomatoes, coconut aminos, okra, and tomato sauce, bring to a simmer and cook for 15 minutes. Sprinkle with fresh parsley to serve.
Per serving: Cal 314, Net Carbs 7g, Fat 25g, Protein 16g

Brazilian Moqueca (Shrimp Stew)

Ingredients for 6 servings
1 ½ pounds shrimp, peeled and deveined
1 cup coconut milk
2 tbsp lime juice
¼ cup diced roasted peppers
3 tbsp olive oil
1 garlic clove, minced
14 ounces diced tomatoes
2 tbsp harissa sauce
1 chopped onion
¼ cup chopped cilantro
Salt and black pepper to taste

Directions and Total Time: approx. 25 minutes
Warm olive oil in a pot and sauté onion and garlic for 3 minutes. Add in tomatoes and shrimp. Cook for 3-4 minutes. Stir in harissa sauce, roasted peppers, and coconut milk and cook for 2 minutes. Add in lime juice and season with salt and pepper. Top with cilantro to serve.
Per serving: Cal 324; Net Carbs 5g; Fats 21g; Protein 23g

Yellow Squash Duck Breast Stew

Ingredients for 2 servings
1 pound duck breast, skin on and sliced
2 yellow squash, sliced
1 tbsp coconut oil
1 green onion bunch, chopped
1 carrot, chopped
2 green bell peppers, chopped
Salt and black pepper, to taste

Directions and Total Time: approx. 20 minutes
Set a pan over high heat and warm oil, stir in the green onions, and cook for 2 minutes. Place in the yellow squash, bell peppers, pepper, salt, and carrot, and cook for 10 minutes. Set another pan over high heat, add in duck slices and cook each side for 3 minutes. Pour the mixture into the vegetable pan. Cook for 3 minutes. Serve.
Per serving: Cal 433; Net Carbs 8g; Fat 21g, Protein 53g

Herby Chicken Stew

Ingredients for 6 servings
2 tbsp butter
2 shallots, finely chopped
2 garlic cloves, minced
1 cup chicken broth
1 tsp dried rosemary
1 tsp dried thyme
1 lb chicken breasts, cubed
1 celery, chopped
1 carrot, chopped
1 bay leaf
1 chili pepper, chopped
2 tomatoes, chopped
Salt black pepper to taste
½ tsp paprika

Directions and Total Time: approx. 60 minutes
Melt butter in a pot over medium heat. Add in shallots, garlic, celery, carrot, salt, and pepper and sauté until tender, about 5 minutes. Pour in chicken broth, rosemary, thyme, chicken breasts, bay leaf, tomatoes, paprika, and chili pepper; bring to a boil. Reduce the heat to low. Simmer for 50 minutes. Discard the bay leaf and adjust the seasoning. Serve warm.
Per serving: Cal 240; Net Carbs 5g; Fat 9.6g, Protein 245

LUNCH & DINNER
Zoodle Bolognese

Ingredients for 4 servings
3 oz olive oil
1 white onion, chopped
1 garlic clove, minced
3 oz carrots, chopped
3 cups crumbled tofu
2 tbsp tomato paste
1 ½ cups crushed tomatoes
Salt and black pepper to taste
1 tbsp dried basil
1 tbsp Worcestershire sauce
2 lbs zucchini, spiralized
2 tbsp vegan butter

Directions and Total Time: approx. 45 minutes
Heat olive oil in a saucepan and sauté onion, garlic, and carrots for 3 minutes. Pour in tofu, tomato paste, tomatoes, salt, pepper, basil, some water, and Worcestershire sauce. Stir and cook for 15 minutes. Melt vegan butter in a skillet and toss in zoodles quickly, about 1 minute. Season with salt and pepper. Serve zoodles topped with the sauce.
Per serving: Cal 425; Net Carbs 6g; Fat 33g; Protein 20g

Baked Tofu with Roasted Peppers

Ingredients for 4 servings
3 oz dairy-free cream cheese
¾ cup vegan mayonnaise
2 oz cucumber, diced
1 large tomato, chopped
Salt and black pepper to taste
2 tsp dried parsley
4 orange bell peppers
2 ½ cups cubed tofu
1 tbsp melted vegan butter
1 tsp dried basil

Directions and Total Time: approx. 20 minutes
Preheat a broiler to 450 F and line a baking sheet with parchment paper. In a salad bowl, combine cream cheese, vegan mayonnaise, cucumber, tomato, salt, pepper, and parsley; refrigerate. Arrange bell peppers and tofu on the paper-lined baking sheet, drizzle with melted butter, and season with basil, salt, and pepper. Use hands to rub the ingredients until evenly coated. Bake for 15 minutes until the peppers have charred lightly and the tofu browned.
Per serving: Cal 840; Net Carbs 8g; Fat 76g; Protein 28g

Spicy Cheese with Tofu Balls

Ingredients for 4 servings
1/3 cup vegan mayonnaise
¼ cup pickled jalapenos
1 tsp paprika powder
1 tbsp mustard powder
1 pinch cayenne pepper
4 oz grated vegan cheddar
1 tbsp flax seed powder
2 ½ cup crumbled tofu
Salt and black pepper to taste
2 tbsp vegan butter, for frying

Directions and Total Time: approx. 40 minutes
In a bowl, mix mayonnaise, jalapenos, paprika, mustard, cayenne, and cheddar; set aside. In another bowl, combine flax seed powder with 3 tbsp water and allow absorbing for 5 minutes. Add the flax egg to the cheese mixture, crumbled tofu, salt, and pepper; mix well. Form meatballs out of the mix. Melt vegan butter in a skillet over medium heat and fry balls until cooked and browned on the outside.
Per serving: Cal 650; Net Carbs 2g; Fat 52g; Protein 43g

Zucchini Boats with Vegan Cheese

Ingredients for 2 servings
1 zucchini, halved
4 tbsp vegan butter
2 garlic cloves, minced
1½ oz baby kale
Salt and black pepper to taste
2 tbsp tomato sauce
1 cup vegan cheese
1 tbsp olive oil

Directions and Total Time: approx. 40 minutes
Preheat oven to 375 F. Scoop out zucchini pulp with a spoon. Keep the flesh. Grease a baking sheet with cooking spray and place the zucchini boats on top. Melt butter in a skillet and sauté garlic until fragrant and slightly browned, 4 minutes. Add in kale and zucchini pulp. Cook until the kale wilts; season with salt and pepper. Spoon tomato sauce into the boats and spread to coat evenly. Spoon kale mixture into the zucchinis and sprinkle with vegan cheese. Bake for 25 minutes. Drizzle with olive oil.
Per serving: Cal 620; Net Carbs 4g; Fat 57g; Protein 20g

Sweet & Spicy Brussel Sprout Stir-Fry

Ingredients for 4 servings
4 tbsp butter
4 shallots, chopped
1 tbsp apple cider vinegar
Salt and black pepper to taste
2 cups Brussels sprouts, halved
Hot chili sauce

Directions and Total Time: approx. 15 minutes
Melt half of butter in a saucepan over medium heat and sauté shallots for 2 minutes until slightly soften. Add in apple cider vinegar, salt, and pepper. Stir and reduce the heat to cook the shallots further with continuous stirring, about 5 minutes. Transfer to a plate. Pour Brussel sprouts into the saucepan and stir-fry with remaining vegan butter until softened. Season with salt and pepper, stir in the shallots and hot chili sauce, and heat for a few seconds.

Per serving: Cal 260; Net Carbs 7g; Fat 23g; Protein 3g

Roasted Butternut Squash with Chimichurri

Ingredients for 4 servings
Zest and juice of 1 lemon
½ red bell pepper, chopped
1 jalapeño pepper, chopped
1 cup olive oil
½ cup chopped fresh parsley
2 garlic cloves, minced
Salt and black pepper to taste
1 lb butternut squash
1 tbsp butter, melted
3 tbsp toasted pine nuts

Directions and Total Time: approx. 15 minutes
In a bowl, add lemon zest and juice, bell pepper, jalapeño, olive oil, parsley, garlic, salt, and pepper. Use an immersion blender to grind the ingredients until desired consistency is achieved; set chimichurri aside. Slice the squash into rounds and remove the seeds. Drizzle with butter and season with salt and pepper. Preheat grill pan over medium heat and cook the squash for 2 minutes on each side. Scatter pine nuts on top and serve with chimichurri.

Per serving: Cal 650; Net Carbs 6g; Fat 44g; Protein 55g

Tofu Eggplant Pizza

Ingredients for 4 servings

2 eggplants, sliced
1/3 cup melted butter
2 garlic cloves, minced
1 red onion
12 oz crumbled tofu
7 oz tomato sauce
Salt and black pepper to taste
½ tsp cinnamon powder
1 cup grated Parmesan
¼ cup chopped fresh oregano

Directions and Total Time: approx. 45 minutes

Preheat oven to 400 F and line a baking sheet with parchment paper. Brush eggplants with butter. Bake until lightly browned, 20 minutes. Heat the remaining butter in a skillet and sauté garlic and onion until fragrant and soft, about 3 minutes. Stir in tofu and cook for 3 minutes. Add tomato sauce and season with salt and pepper. Simmer for 10 minutes. Remove eggplants from the oven and spread the tofu sauce on top. Sprinkle with Parmesan cheese and oregano. Bake further for 10 minutes.

Per serving: Cal 600; Net Carbs 12g; Fat 46g; Protein 26g

Tomato Artichoke Pizza

Ingredients for 4 servings

2 oz canned artichokes, cut into wedges
2 tbsp flax seed powder
4¼ oz grated broccoli
6¼ oz grated Parmesan
½ tsp salt
2 tbsp tomato sauce
2 oz mozzarella cheese, grated
1 garlic clove, thinly sliced
1 tbsp dried oregano
Green olives for garnish

Directions and Total Time: approx. 40 minutes

Preheat oven to 350 F and line a baking sheet with parchment paper. In a bowl, mix flax seed powder and 6 tbsp water and allow thickening for 5 minutes. When the flax egg is ready, add broccoli, 4 ½ ounces of Parmesan cheese, salt, and stir to combine. Pour the mixture into the baking sheet and bake until the crust is lightly browned, 20 minutes. Remove from oven and spread tomato sauce on top, sprinkle with the remaining Parmesan and mozzarella cheeses, add artichokes and garlic. Spread oregano on top. Bake pizza for 10 minutes at 420 F. Garnish with olives.

Per serving: Cal 860; Net Carbs 10g; Fat 63g; Protein 55g

White Pizza with Mixed Mushrooms

Ingredients for 4 servings
2 tbsp flax seed powder
½ cup mayonnaise
¾ cup almond flour
1 tbsp psyllium husk powder
1 tsp baking powder
2 oz mixed mushrooms, sliced
1 tbsp basil pesto
2 tbsp olive oil
½ cup coconut cream
¾ cup grated Parmesan

Directions and Total Time: approx. 35 minutes
Preheat oven to 350 F. Combine flax seed powder with 6 tbsp water and allow sitting for 5 minutes. Whisk in mayonnaise, flour, psyllium husk, baking powder, and ½ tsp salt; let rest. Pour batter into a baking sheet.
Bake for 10 minutes. In a bowl, mix mushrooms with pesto, olive oil, salt, and pepper. Remove crust from the oven and spread coconut cream on top. Add the mushroom mixture and Parmesan. Bake the pizza further until the cheese melts, about 5-10 minutes. Slice and serve.
Per serving: Cal 750; Net Carbs 6g; Fat 69g; Protein 22g

Pepperoni Fat Head Pizza

Ingredients for 4 servings
3 ½ cups grated mozzarella
2 tbsp cream cheese, softened
2 eggs, beaten
1/3 cup almond flour
1 tsp dried oregano
½ cup sliced pepperoni

Directions and Total Time: approx. 35 minutes
Preheat oven to 420 F and line a round pizza pan with parchment paper. Microwave 2 cups of the mozzarella cheese and cream cheese for 1 minute. Mix in eggs and almond flour. Transfer the pizza "dough" onto a flat surface and knead until smooth. Spread it on the pizza pan. Bake for 6 minutes. Top with remaining mozzarella, oregano, and pepperoni. Bake for 15 minutes.
Per serving: Cal 229; Net Carbs 0.4g; Fats 7g; Protein 36.4g

Vegan Cordon Bleu Casserole

Ingredients for 4 servings
2 cups grilled tofu, cubed
1 cup smoked seitan, cubed
1 cup cream cheese
1 tbsp mustard powder
1 tbsp plain vinegar
1 ¼ cup grated cheddar
½ cup baby spinach
4 tbsp olive oil

Directions and Total Time: approx. 30 minutes
Preheat oven to 400 F. Mix cream cheese, mustard powder, plain vinegar, and cheddar in a baking dish. Top with tofu and seitan. Bake until the casserole is golden brown, about 20 minutes. Drizzle with olive oil.
Per serving: Cal 980; Net Carbs 6g; Fat 92g; Protein 30g

Parmesan Meatballs

Ingredients for 4 servings
½ lb ground beef
½ lb ground Italian sausage
¾ cup pork rinds
½ cup grated Parmesan cheese
2 eggs
1 tsp onion powder
1 tsp garlic powder
1 tbsp chopped fresh basil
Salt and black pepper to taste
2 tsp dried Italian seasoning
3 tbsp olive oil
2 ½ cups marinara sauce

Directions and Total Time: approx. 1 hour
In a bowl, add beef, Italian sausage, pork rinds, Parmesan cheese, eggs, onion powder, garlic powder, basil, salt, pepper, and Italian seasoning. Form meatballs out of the mixture. Heat the remaining olive oil in a skillet and brown the meatballs for 10 minutes. Pour in marinara sauce and submerge the meatballs in the sauce; cook for 45 minutes.
Per serving: Cal 513; Net Carbs 8.2g; Fat 24g; Protein 35g

Seitan Cauliflower Gratin

Ingredients for 4 servings
2 oz butter
1 leek, coarsely chopped
1 onion, coarsely chopped
2 cups broccoli florets
1 cup cauliflower florets
2 cups crumbled seitan
1 cup coconut cream
2 tbsp mustard powder
5 oz grated Parmesan
4 tbsp fresh rosemary

Directions and Total Time: approx. 40 minutes
Preheat oven to 450 F. Put half of butter in a pot, set over medium heat to melt. Add leek, onion, broccoli, and cauliflower and cook until the vegetables have softened, about 6 minutes. Transfer them to a baking dish. Melt the remaining butter in a skillet over medium heat, and cook seitan until browned.
Mix coconut cream and mustard powder in a bowl. Pour the mixture over the veggies. Scatter seitan and Parmesan on top and sprinkle with rosemary. Bake for 15 minutes. Serve warm.
Per serving: Cal 480; Net Carbs 9.8g; Fat 40g; Protein 16g

Walnut Stuffed Mushrooms

Ingredients for 4 servings
½ cup grated Pecorino Romano cheese
12 button mushrooms, stemmed
¼ cup pork rinds
2 garlic cloves, minced
2 tbsp chopped fresh parsley
Salt and black pepper to taste
¼ cup ground walnuts
¼ cup olive oil

Directions and Total Time: approx. 30 minutes
Preheat oven to 400 F. In a bowl, mix pork rinds, Pecorino Romano cheese, garlic, parsley, salt, and pepper. Brush a baking sheet with 2 tablespoons of the olive oil. Spoon the cheese mixture into the mushrooms and arrange on the baking sheet. Top with the ground walnuts and drizzle the remaining olive oil on the mushrooms. Bake for 20 minutes or until golden. Transfer to a platter and serve.
Per serving: Cal 292; Net Carbs 7.1g; Fat 25g; Protein 8g

POULTRY

Chicken with Tomato and Zucchini

Ingredients for 4 servings
2 tbsp ghee
1 lb chicken thighs
2 cloves garlic, minced
1 (14 oz) can whole tomatoes
1 zucchini, diced
10 fresh basil leaves, chopped

Directions and Total Time: approx. 45 minutes
Melt ghee in a saucepan, season the chicken with salt and pepper, and fry for 4 minutes on each side. Remove to a plate. Sauté garlic in the ghee for 2 minutes, pour in tomatoes, and cook for 8 minutes. Add in zucchini and cook for 4 minutes. Season the sauce with salt and pepper, stir, and add the chicken. Coat with sauce and simmer for 3 minutes. Serve chicken with sauce garnished with basil.

Per serving: Cal 468, Net Carbs 2g, Fat 39g, Protein 26g

Cauli Rice & Chicken Collard Wraps

Ingredients for 4 servings
2 tbsp avocado oil
1 large yellow onion, chopped
2 garlic cloves, minced
Salt and black pepper to taste
1 jalapeño pepper, chopped
1 ½ lb chicken breasts, cubed
1 cup cauliflower rice
2 tsp hot sauce
8 collard leaves
¼ cup crème fraiche

Directions and Total Time: approx. 30 minutes
Heat avocado oil in a deep skillet and sauté onion and garlic until softened, 3 minutes. Stir in jalapeño pepper salt, and pepper. Mix in chicken and cook until no longer pink on all sides, 10 minutes. Add in cauliflower rice and hot sauce. Sauté until the cauliflower slightly softens, 3 minutes. Lay out the collards on a clean flat surface and spoon the curried mixture onto the middle part of the leaves, about 3 tbsp per leaf. Spoon crème fraiche on top, wrap the leaves, and serve immediately.

Per serving: Cal 437; Net Carbs 1.8g; Fat 28g; Protein 38g

Almond Crusted Chicken Zucchini Stacks

Ingredients for 4 servings
1 ½ lb chicken thighs, skinless and boneless, cut into strips
3 tbsp almond flour
Salt and black pepper to taste
2 large zucchinis, sliced
4 tbsp olive oil
2 tsp Italian mixed herb blend
½ cup chicken broth

Directions and Total Time: approx. 30 minutes
Preheat oven to 400 F. In a zipper bag, add almond flour, salt, and pepper. Mix and add the chicken slices. Seal the bag and shake to coat. Arrange the zucchinis on a greased baking sheet. Season with salt and pepper, and drizzle with 2 tbsp of olive oil. Remove the chicken from the almond flour mixture, shake off, and put 2-3 chicken strips on each zucchini. Season with herb blend and drizzle again with olive oil. Bake for 8 minutes; remove the sheet and pour in broth. Bake further for 10 minutes. Serve warm.
Per serving: Cal 512; Net Carbs 1.2g; Fat 42g; Protein 29g

Paleo Coconut Flour Chicken Nuggets

Ingredients for 2 servings
½ cup coconut flour
1 egg
2 tbsp garlic powder
2 chicken breasts, cubed
Salt and black pepper, to taste
½ cup butter

Directions and Total Time: approx. 30 minutes
In a bowl, combine salt, garlic powder, flour, and pepper, and stir. In a separate bowl, beat the egg. Add the chicken in egg mixture, then in the flour mixture. Set a pan over medium heat and warm butter. Add in chicken nuggets, and cook for 6 minutes on each side. Remove to paper towels, drain the excess grease and serve.
Per serving: Cal 417, Net Carbs 4.3g, Fat 37g, Protein 35g

Bacon Chicken Skillet with Bok Choy

Ingredients for 4 servings
2 lb ground chicken, cubed
Salt and black pepper to taste
4 bacon slices, chopped
1 tbsp coconut oil
1 orange bell pepper, chopped
2 cups baby bok choy
2 tbsp chopped oregano
2 garlic cloves, pressed

Directions and Total Time: approx. 30 minutes
Season the chicken with salt and pepper; set aside. Heat a skillet over medium heat and fry bacon until brown and crispy. Transfer to a plate. Melt coconut oil in the skillet and cook chicken until no longer pink, 10 minutes. Remove to the bacon plate. Add bell pepper and bok choy and sauté until softened, 5 minutes. Stir in bacon, chicken, oregano, and garlic, for 3 minutes. Serve with cauli rice.
Per serving: Cal 639; Net Carbs 1.2g; Fat 48g; Protein 46g

Celery Chicken Sausage Frittata

Ingredients for 4 servings
12 whole eggs
1 cup crème fraiche
2 tbsp butter
1 celery stalk, chopped
12 oz ground chicken sausages
¼ cup shredded Swiss cheese

Directions and Total Time: approx. 45 minutes
Preheat oven to 350 F. In a bowl, whisk eggs, crème fraiche, salt, and pepper. Melt butter in a safe oven skillet over medium heat. Sauté celery until soft, 5 minutes; set aside. Add the sausages to the skillet and cook until brown with frequent stirring to break the lumps that form, 8 minutes. Scatter celery on top, pour the egg mixture all over, and sprinkle with Swiss cheese. Put the skillet in the oven and bake until the eggs set and cheese melts, 20 minutes. Slice the frittata, and serve warm.
Per serving: Cal 529; Net Carbs 3g; Fat 44g; Protein 28g

Rosemary Turkey Brussels Sprouts Cakes

Ingredients for 4 servings
For the burgers
1 pound ground turkey
1 egg
1 onion, chopped
1 garlic clove, minced
1 tsp fresh rosemary, chopped
4 tbsp olive oil
For the fried Brussels sprouts
1 ½ lb Brussels sprouts
4 tbsp olive oil
2 tbsp balsamic vinegar
Salt to taste

Directions and Total Time: approx. 35 minutes
Preheat oven to 320 F and arrange Brussels sprouts in a baking dish. Toss to coat with olive oil and season with salt. Bake for 20 minutes, stirring once. Pour vinegar over and cook for 5 minutes. Combine burger ingredients in a bowl. Form patties out of the mixture. Set a pan, warm olive oil, and fry patties until cooked through. Serve.
Per serving: Cal 535; Net Carbs 6.7g; Fat 38g; Protein 31g

Grilled Garlic Chicken with Cauliflower

Ingredients for 6 servings
1 head cauliflower, cut into florets
3 tbsp smoked paprika
2 tsp garlic powder
1 tbsp olive oil
6 chicken breasts

Directions and Total Time: approx. 30 minutes
Place the cauliflower florets onto the steamer basket over boiling water and steam for approximately 8 minutes or until crisp-tender; set aside. Grease grill grate with cooking spray and preheat to 400 F. Combine paprika, salt, black pepper, and garlic powder in a bowl. Brush chicken with olive oil and sprinkle spice mixture over and massage with hands. Grill chicken for 7 minutes per side until well-cooked, and plate. Serve warm.
Per serving: Cal 422, Net Carbs 2g, Fat 35g, Protein 26g

Cucumber Salsa Topped Turkey Patties

Ingredients for 4 servings
2 spring onions, thinly sliced
1 pound ground turkey
1 egg
4 garlic cloves, minced
1 tbsp chopped herbs
2 tbsp ghee
1 tbsp apple cider vinegar
1 tbsp chopped dill
2 cucumbers, grated
1 cup sour cream
1 jalapeño pepper, minced
2 tbsp olive oil

Directions and Total Time: approx. 30 minutes
In a bowl, place spring onions, turkey, egg, two garlic cloves, and herbs; mix to combine. Make patties out of the mixture. Melt ghee in a skillet over medium heat. Cook the patties for 3 minutes per side. In a bowl, combine vinegar, dill, remaining garlic, cucumber, sour cream, jalapeño, and olive oil; toss well. Serve patties topped with salsa.
Per serving: Cal 475; Net Carbs 5g; Fat 38g; Protein 26g

Turkey with Avocado Sauce

Ingredients for 4 servings
1 avocado, pitted
½ cup mayonnaise
3 tbsp ghee
1 pound turkey breasts
1 cup chopped cilantro leaves
½ cup chicken broth

Directions and Total Time: approx. 25 minutes
Spoon avocado, mayo, and salt into a food processor and puree until smooth. Season with salt. Pour sauce into a jar and refrigerate.
Melt ghee in a skillet, fry turkey for 4 minutes on each side. Remove to a plate. Pour broth in the same skillet and add cilantro. Bring to a simmer for 15 minutes and add the turkey. Cook on low heat for 5 minutes until liquid reduces by half. Dish and spoon mayo-avocado sauce over.
Per serving: Cal 398, Net Carbs 4g, Fat 32g, Protein 24g

Bell Pepper Turkey Keto Carnitas

Ingredients for 4 servings
1 lb turkey breasts, sliced
1 garlic clove, minced
1 red onion, sliced
1 green chili, minced
2 tsp ground cumin
2 tbsp lime juice
1 tsp sweet paprika
2 tbsp olive oil
1 tsp ground coriander
1 green bell pepper, sliced
1 red bell pepper, sliced
1 tbsp fresh cilantro, chopped

Directions and Total Time: approx. 25 minutes
In a bowl, combine lime juice, cumin, garlic, coriander, paprika, salt, green chili, and pepper. Toss in the turkey pieces to coat well. Place a pan over medium heat and warm oil. Cook in turkey on each side, for 3 minutes; set aside. In the same pan, sauté bell peppers, cilantro, and onion for 6 minutes. Serve keto carnitas in lettuce leaves.
Per serving: Cal 262; Net Carbs 4.2g; Fat 15.2g; Protein 26g

Caprese Turkey Meatballs

Ingredients for 4 servings
2 tbsp chopped sun-dried tomatoes
1 pound ground turkey
2 tbsp chopped basil
½ tsp garlic powder
1 egg
¼ cup almond flour
2 tbsp olive oil
½ cup shredded mozzarella
Salt and black pepper to taste

Directions and Total Time: approx. 15 minutes
Place everything except for the oil in a bowl; mix well. Form 16 meatballs out of the mixture. Heat the olive oil in a skillet. Cook the meatballs for about 6 minutes. Serve.
Per serving: Cal 310; Net Carbs 2g; Fat 26g; Protein 22g

Tasty Curried Chicken Meatballs

Ingredients for 4 servings
3 lb ground chicken
1 yellow onion, chopped
2 green bell peppers, chopped
3 garlic cloves, minced
2 tbsp melted butter
1 tsp dried parsley
2 tbsp hot sauce
Salt and black pepper to taste
1 tbsp red curry powder
3 tbsp olive oil

Directions and Total Time: approx. 30 minutes
Preheat oven to 400 F. In a bowl, combine chicken, onion, bell peppers, garlic, butter, parsley, hot sauce, salt, pepper, and curry. Form meatballs and place on a greased baking sheet. Drizzle with olive oil and bake until the meatballs brown on the outside and cook within, 25 minutes. Serve.
Per serving: Cal 908; Net Carbs 2.7g; Fat 67g; Protein 65g

Hot Chicken Meatball Tray

Ingredients for 4 servings
1 egg
1 pound ground chicken
Salt and black pepper, to taste
1 red pepper, chopped
2 spring onions, chopped
¼ cup Pecorino, grated
1 tbsp dry Italian seasoning
2 tbsp olive oil
¼ cup hot sauce
2 tbsp parsley, chopped

Directions and Total Time: approx. 25 minutes
Preheat oven to 480 F. In a bowl, combine ground chicken, red pepper, onions, Italian seasoning, Pecorino cheese, salt, black pepper, parsley, and egg, and mix well with hands. Form into meatballs, arrange them on a greased with olive oil baking tray and bake for 16 minutes. Remove from the oven to a bowl and cover with hot sauce. Serve.
Per serving: Cal 383; Net Carbs 4.4g; Fat 28.1g; Protein 26g

Creamy Turkey & Broccoli Bake

Ingredients for 4 servings
1 lb turkey breasts, cooked
2 tbsp butter, melted
1 head broccoli, cut into florets
½ cup buttermilk
1 carrot, sliced
½ cup heavy cream
1 cup cheddar cheese, grated
4 tbsp pork rinds, crushed
Salt and black pepper, to taste
1 tsp oregano

Directions and Total Time: approx. 40 minutes
Cook broccoli in salted water for 4 minutes. Shred the turkey and place into a bowl together with buttermilk, butter, oregano, carrot, and broccoli; mix to combine. Season with salt and pepper, and transfer the mixture to a greased pan. Pour in heavy cream and top with cheese. Cover with pork rinds. Bake for 25 minutes at 450 F.
Per serving: Cal 469; Net Carbs 6.2g; Fat 3g; Protein 38.4g

Cheesy Turkey Sausage Egg Cups

Ingredients for 4 servings
1 cup Pecorino Romano cheese, grated
1 tsp butter
6 eggs
Salt and black pepper, to taste
½ tsp dried thyme
3 turkey sausages, chopped

Directions and Total Time: approx. 15 minutes
Preheat oven to 400 F and grease muffin cups with cooking spray.
In a skillet over medium heat add the butter and cook the turkey sausages for 4-5 minutes. Beat 3 eggs with a fork. Add in sausages, cheese, and seasonings. Divide between the ups and bake for 4 minutes. Crack in an egg to each of the cups. Bake for an additional 4 minutes. Allow cooling before serving.
Per serving: Cal 423; Net Carbs 2.2g; Fat 34g; Protein 26.4g

BEEF

Classic Beef Ragu with Veggie Pasta

Ingredients for 4 servings
8 mixed bell peppers, spiralized
2 tbsp butter
1 lb ground beef
Salt and black pepper to taste
¼ cup tomato sauce
1 small red onion, spiralized
1 cup grated Parmesan cheese

Directions and Total Time: approx. 20 minutes
Heat the butter in a skillet and cook the beef until brown, 5 minutes. Season with salt and pepper. Stir in tomato sauce and cook for 10 minutes, until the sauce reduces by a quarter. Stir in bell peppers and onion noodles; cook for 1 minute. Top with Parmesan cheese and serve.
Per serving: Cal 451; Net Carbs 7.2g; Fats 25g; Protein 40g

Barbecued Beef Pizza

Ingredients for 4 servings
1 cup grated mozzarella cheese
1 ½ cups grated Gruyere cheese
1 lb ground beef
2 eggs, beaten
¼ cup sugar-free BBQ sauce
¼ cup sliced red onion
2 bacon slices, chopped
2 tbsp chopped parsley

Directions and Total Time: approx. 40 minutes
Preheat oven to 390 F and line a round pizza pan with parchment paper. Mix beef, mozzarella cheese and eggs, and salt. Spread the pizza "dough" on the pan and bake for 20 minutes. Spread BBQ sauce on top, scatter Gruyere cheese all over, followed by the red onion, and bacon slices. Bake for 15 minutes or until the cheese has melted and the back is crispy. Serve warm sprinkled with parsley.
Per serving: Cal 538; Net Carbs 0.4g; Fats 32g; Protein 56g

Beef with Parsnip Noodles

Ingredients for 4 servings
1 lb beef stew meat, cut into strips
1 cup sun-dried tomatoes in oil, chopped
1 cup shaved Parmesan cheese
3 tbsp butter
Salt and black pepper to taste
4 large parsnips, spiralized
4 garlic cloves, minced
1 ¼ cups heavy cream
¼ tsp dried basil
¼ tsp red chili flakes
2 tbsp chopped parsley

Directions and Total Time: approx. 35 minutes
Melt butter in a skillet and sauté the parsnips until softened, 5-7 minutes. Set aside. Season the beef with salt and pepper and add to the same skillet; cook until brown, and cooked within, 8-10 minutes. Stir in sun-dried tomatoes and garlic and cook until fragrant, 1 minute. Reduce the heat to low and stir in heavy cream and Parmesan cheese. Simmer until the cheese melts. Season with basil and red chili flakes. Fold in the parsnips until well coated and cook for 2 more minutes. Garnish with parsley and serve.
Per serving: Cal 596; Net Carbs 6.5g; Fats 35g; Protein 37g

Assorted Grilled Veggies & Beef Steaks

Ingredients for 4 servings
1 red and 1 green bell peppers, cut into strips
4 tbsp olive oil
1 ¼ pounds sirloin steaks
Salt and black pepper to taste
3 tbsp balsamic vinegar
½ lb asparagus, trimmed
1 eggplant, sliced
2 zucchinis, sliced
1 red onion, sliced

Directions and Total Time: approx. 30 minutes
Divide the meat and vegetables between 2 bowls. Mix salt, pepper, olive oil, and balsamic vinegar in a 2 bowl. Rub the beef all over with half of this mixture. Pour the remaining mixture over the vegetables. Preheat a grill pan. Drain the steaks and reserve the marinade. Sear the steaks on both sides for 10 minutes, flipping once halfway through; set aside. Pour the vegetables and marinade in the pan; and cook for 5 minutes, turning once. Serve.
Per serving: Cal 459; Net Carbs 4.5g; Fat 31g; Protein 32.8g

Classic Swedish Coconut Meatballs

Ingredients for 4 servings
1 ½ lb ground beef
2 tsp garlic powder
1 tsp onion powder
Salt and black pepper to taste
2 tbsp olive oil
2 tbsp butter
2 tbsp almond flour
1 cup beef broth
½ cup coconut cream
¼ freshly chopped dill
¼ cup chopped parsley

Directions and Total Time: approx. 30 minutes
Preheat oven to 400 F. In a bowl, combine beef, garlic powder, onion powder, salt, and pepper. Form meatballs from the mixture and place on a greased baking sheet. Drizzle with olive oil and bake until the meat cooks, 10-15 minutes. Remove the baking sheet. Melt butter in a saucepan and stir in almond flour until smooth. Gradually mix in broth, while stirring until thickened, 2 minutes. Stir in coconut cream and dill, simmer for 1 minute and stir in meatballs. Spoon the meatballs with sauce onto a serving platter and garnish with parsley. Serve immediately.
Per serving: Cal 459; Net Carbs 3.2g; Fat 32g; Protein 40g

Herbed Bolognese Sauce

Ingredients for 5 servings
1 pound ground beef
2 garlic cloves
1 onion, chopped
1 tsp oregano
1 tsp marjoram
1 tsp rosemary
7 oz canned chopped tomatoes
1 tbsp olive oil

Directions and Total Time: approx. 35 minutes
Heat olive oil in a saucepan. Cook onions and garlic for 3 minutes. Add beef and cook until browned, about 5 minutes. Stir in herbs and tomatoes. Cook for 15 minutes.
Per serving: Cal 318; Net Carbs 9g; Fat 20g; Protein 26g

Cheese & Beef Bake

Ingredients for 6 servings
2 lb ground beef
Salt and black pepper to taste
1 cup cauli rice
2 cups chopped cabbage
14 oz can diced tomatoes
1 cup shredded Gouda cheese
Directions and Total Time: approx. 30 minutes
Preheat oven to 370 F. Put beef in a pot, season with salt and pepper, and cook for 6 minutes. Add cauli rice, cabbage, tomatoes, and ¼ cup water. Stir and bring to boil for 5 minutes to thicken the sauce. Spoon the beef mixture into a greased baking dish. Sprinkle with cheese and bake for 15 minutes. Cool for 4 minutes and serve.
Per serving: Cal 385, Net Carbs 5g, Fat 25g, Protein 20g

Beef Burgers with Roasted Brussels Sprouts

Ingredients for 4 servings
1 ½ lb Brussels sprouts, halved
1 pound ground beef
1 egg
½ onion, chopped
1 tsp dried thyme
4 oz butter
Salt and black pepper to taste
Directions and Total Time: approx. 30 minutes
Combine beef, egg, onion, thyme, salt, and pepper in a mixing bowl. Create patties out of the mixture. Set a pan over medium heat, warm half of the butter, and fry the patties until browned. Remove to a plate and cover with aluminium foil. Fry Brussels sprouts in the remaining butter, season to taste, then set into a bowl. Plate the burgers and Brussels sprouts and serve.
Per serving: Cal: 443, Net Carbs: 5g, Fat: 25g, Protein: 31g

Easy Rump Steak Salad

Ingredients for 4 servings
1 pound flank steak
½ pound Brussels sprouts
3 green onions, sliced
1 cucumber, sliced
1 cup green beans, sliced
9 oz mixed salad greens
Salad Dressing
2 tsp Dijon mustard
1 tsp xylitol
3 tbsp extra virgin olive oil
1 tbsp red wine vinegar

Directions and Total Time: approx. 40 minutes
Preheat a grill pan, season the meat with salt and pepper, and brown the steak for 5 minutes per side. Remove to a chopping board and slice thinly. Put Brussels sprouts on a baking sheet, drizzle with olive oil and bake for 25 minutes at 400 F; set aside. In a bowl, mix mustard, xylitol, salt, pepper, vinegar, and olive oil. Set aside. In a shallow salad bowl, add green onions, cucumber, green beans, cooled Brussels sprouts, salad greens, and steak slices. Serve.
Per serving: Cal 244; Net Carbs 3.3g; Fat 11g; Protein 27.4g

Steak Carnitas

Ingredients for 4 servings
2 lb sirloin steak, cut into strips
2 tbsp Cajun seasoning
4 oz guacamole
Salt to taste
2 tbsp olive oil
2 shallots, sliced
1 red bell pepper, sliced
8 low carb tortillas

Directions and Total Time: approx. 35 minutes
Preheat grill to 425 F. Rub the steaks all over with Cajun seasoning and place in the fridge for 1 hour. Grill the steaks for 6 minutes per side, flipping once. Wrap in foil and let sit for 10 minutes. Heat olive oil in a skillet and sauté shallots and bell pepper for 5 minutes. Share the strips in the tortillas and top with veggies and guacamole.
Per serving: Cal 381; Net Carbs 5g; Fat 16.7g; Protein 47g

Tasty Beef Cheeseburgers

Ingredients for 4 servings
1 lb ground beef
1 tsp dried parsley
½ tsp Worcestershire sauce
Salt and black pepper to taste
1 cup feta cheese, shredded
4 zero carb buns, halved

Directions and Total Time: approx. 20 minutes
Preheat grill to 400 F and grease the grate with cooking spray. Mix beef, parsley, Worcestershire sauce, salt, and pepper with until evenly combined. Make patties out of the mixture. Cook on the grill for 7 minutes one side. Flip the patties and top with cheese. Cook for another 7 minutes. Remove the patties and sandwich into 2 halves of a bun each. Serve with a tomato dipping sauce.
Per serving: Cal 386, Net Carbs 2g, Fat 32g, Protein 21g

Beef & Pesto Filled Tomatoes

Ingredients for 6 servings
1 tbsp olive oil
¼ lb ground beef
Salt and black pepper to taste
4 medium tomatoes, halved
4 tsp basil pesto
5 tbsp shredded Parmesan

Directions and Total Time: approx. 30 minutes
Preheat oven to 400 F. Heat olive oil in a skillet, add in beef, season with salt and pepper, and cook until brown while breaking the lumps that form, 8 minutes. Remove the seeds of tomatoes to create a cavity and spoon the beef inside them. Top with pesto and Parmesan. Place the filled tomatoes on a greased baking sheet and bake until the cheese melts and the tomatoes slightly brown, 20 minutes.
Per serving: Cal 122; Net Carbs 2.9g; Fat 4.4g; Protein 7.3g

Habanero Beef Cauliflower Pilaf

Ingredients for 4 servings
3 tbsp olive oil
½ lb ground beef
Salt and black pepper to taste
1 yellow onion, chopped
3 garlic cloves, minced
1 habanero pepper, minced
½ tsp Italian seasoning
2 ½ cups cauliflower rice
2 tbsp tomato paste
½ cup beef broth
¼ cup chopped parsley
1 lemon, sliced

Directions and Total Time: approx. 30 minutes
Heat olive oil in a skillet over medium heat and cook the beef until no longer brown, 8 minutes. Season with salt and pepper and spoon into a serving plate. In the same skillet, sauté onion, garlic, and habanero pepper, 2 minutes. Mix in Italian seasoning. Stir in cauli rice, tomato paste, and broth. Season to taste, and cook covered for 10 minutes. Mix in beef for 3 minutes. Garnish with parsley to serve.
Per serving: Cal 216; Net Carbs 3.8g; Fat 14g; Protein 15g

Beef Patties with Cherry Tomatoes

Ingredients for 4 servings
2 slices cheddar cheese, cut into 4 pieces each
2 pearl onions, thinly sliced into 8 pieces
½ lb ground beef
1 tsp garlic powder
1 tsp onion powder
8 slices zero carb bread
2 tbsp ranch dressing
4 cherry tomatoes, halved

Directions and Total Time: approx. 30 minutes
Preheat oven to 400 F. In a bowl, combine beef, salt, pepper, garlic and onion powders. Form 8 patties and place them on a greased baking sheet. Bake until brown and cooked, 10 minutes. Let cool for 3 minutes. Cut out 16 circles from the bread slices. Lay half of the bread circles on clean, flat surface and brush with the ranch dressing. Place the meat patties on the bread slices, divide cheese slices on top, onions, and tomatoes. Cover with the remaining bread slices and secure with a toothpick. Serve.
Per serving: Cal 281; Net Carbs 2.8g; Fat 12g; Protein 20g

Mexican Pizza

Ingredients for 4 servings
2 cups shredded mozzarella
2 tbsp cream cheese, softened
¾ cup almond flour
2 eggs, beaten
¾ lb ground beef
2 tsp taco seasoning mix
Salt and black pepper to taste
½ cup chicken broth
1 ½ cups salsa
2 cups Mexican 4 cheese blend

Directions and Total Time: approx. 50 minutes
Preheat oven to 390 F and line a pizza pan with parchment paper. Microwave 2 cups of mozzarella cheese and cream cheese for 30 seconds. Remove and mix in almond flour and eggs. Spread the mixture on the pizza pan and bake for 15 minutes. Add the beef to a pot and cook for 5 minutes. Stir in taco seasoning, salt, pepper, and chicken broth. Cook for 3 minutes. Stir in salsa. Spread the beef mixture onto the crust and scatter the cheese blend on top. Bake until the cheese melts, 15 minutes. Slice and serve hot.
Per serving: Cal 556; Net Carbs 4.2g; Fats 30g; Protein 59g

Beef with Broccoli Rice & Eggs

Ingredients for 4 servings
2 cups cauli rice
3 cups mixed vegetables
3 tbsp butter
1 lb sirloin steak, sliced
4 fresh eggs
Hot sauce for topping

Directions and Total Time: approx. 25 minutes
Mix cauli rice and mixed vegetables in a bowl, sprinkle with a little water, and steam in the microwave for 1 minute. Share into 4 serving bowls. Melt butter in a skillet, season beef with salt and pepper, and brown for 5 minutes on each side. Ladle the meat onto the vegetables. Crack in an egg, season with salt and pepper and cook for 3 minutes. Remove egg onto the vegetable bowl and fry the remaining 3 eggs. Drizzle beef with hot sauce to serve.
Per serving: Cal 320, Net Carbs 4g, Fat 26g, Protein 15g

Polish Beef Tripe

Ingredients for 6 servings
1 ½ lb beef tripe
4 cups buttermilk
Salt and black pepper to taste
1 parsnip, chopped
2 tsp marjoram
3 tbsp butter
2 large onions, sliced
3 tomatoes, diced

Directions and Total Time: approx. 30 min + cooling time
Put tripe in a bowl and cover with buttermilk. Refrigerate for 3 hours. Remove from buttermilk and season with salt and pepper. Heat 2 tablespoons of butter in a skillet and brown the tripe on both sides for 6 minutes in total; set aside. Add the remaining oil and sauté onions for 3 minutes. Include tomatoes and parsnip, and cook for 15 minutes. Put the tripe in the sauce and cook for 3 minutes.
Per serving: Cal 342, Net Carbs 1g, Fat 27g, Protein 22g

Smoked Paprika Grilled Ribs

Ingredients for 4 servings
4 tbsp sugar-free BBQ sauce + extra for serving
2 tbsp erythritol
Salt and black pepper to taste
1 tbsp olive oil
3 tsp smoked paprika
1 tsp garlic powder
1 lb beef spare ribs

Directions and Total Time: approx. 35 minutes
Mix erythritol, salt, pepper, oil, smoked paprika, and garlic powder. Brush on the meaty sides of the ribs and wrap in foil. Sit for 30 minutes to marinate.
Preheat oven to 400 F, place wrapped ribs on a baking sheet, and cook for 40 minutes. Remove ribs and aluminium foil, brush with BBQ sauce, and brown under the broiler for 10 minutes on both sides. Slice and serve with extra BBQ sauce and lettuce tomato salad.
Per serving: Cal 395; Net Carbs 3g; Fat 33g; Protein 21g

Beef Broccoli Curry

Ingredients for 6 servings
1 head broccoli, cut into florets
1 tbsp olive oil
1 ½ lb ground beef
1 tbsp ginger-garlic paste
1 tsp garam masala
1 (7 oz) can whole tomatoes
Salt and chili pepper to taste

Directions and Total Time: approx. 30 minutes
Heat oil in a saucepan, add beef, ginger-garlic paste and season with garam masala. Cook for 5 minutes. Stir in tomatoes and broccoli, season with salt and chili pepper, and cook for 6 minutes. Add ¼ cup of water and bring to a boil for 10 minutes or until the water has reduced by half. Adjust taste with salt. Spoon into serving bowls and serve.
Per serving: Cal 374, Net Carbs 2g, Fat 33g, Protein 22g

Shitake Butter Steak

Ingredients for 4 servings
2 cups shitake mushrooms, sliced
4 ribeye steaks
2 tbsp butter
2 tsp olive oil
Salt and black pepper to taste

Directions and Total Time: approx. 25 minutes
Heat olive oil in a pan over medium heat. Rub the steaks with salt and pepper and cook for 4 minutes per side. Set aside. Melt butter in the pan and cook the shitakes for 4 minutes. Pour the butter and mushrooms over the steak.
Per serving: Cal 370; Net Carbs 3g; Fat 31g; Protein 33g

Gruyere Beef Burgers with Sweet Onion

Ingredients for 4 servings
4 zero carb hamburger buns, halved
1 medium white onion, sliced
3 tbsp olive oil
2 tbsp balsamic vinegar
2 tsp erythritol
1 lb ground beef
Salt and black pepper to taste
4 slices Gruyere cheese
Mayonnaise to serve

Directions and Total Time: approx. 35 minutes
Heat 2 tbsp of olive oil in a skillet and add onion. Sauté for 15 minutes until golden brown and add erythritol, balsamic vinegar, and salt. Cook for 3 more minutes; set aside.Make 4 patties out of the ground beef and season with salt and pepper. Then, heat the remaining olive oil in a skillet and cook the patties for 4 minutes on each side. Place a Gruyere slice on each patty and top with the caramelized onions. Put the patties with cheese and onions into two halves of the buns. Serve with mayonnaise.
Per serving: Cal 487; Net Carbs 7.8g; Fat 32g; Protein 38g

PORK

Pulled Pork Tenderloin with Avocado

Ingredients for 8 servings
4 pounds pork tenderloin
1 tbsp avocado oil
½ cup chicken stock
¼ cup jerk seasoning
6 avocado, sliced
Salt and black pepper to taste

Directions and Total Time: approx. 2 hours
Rub the pork shoulder with jerk seasoning, and set in a greased baking dish. Pour in the stock, and cook for 1 hour 30 minutes in your oven at 350 F covered with aluminium foil. Discard the foil and cook for another 20 minutes. Leave to rest for 10-15 minutes, and shred it with 2 forks. Serve topped with avocado slices.
Per serving: Cal 567, Net Carbs 4.1g, Fat 42.6g, Protein 42g

Broccoli Tips with Lemon Pork Chops

Ingredients for 6 servings
1 lb fresh broccoli tips, halved
3 tbsp lemon juice
3 cloves garlic, pureed
1 tbsp olive oil
6 pork loin chops
1 tbsp butter
2 tbsp white wine

Directions and Total Time: approx. 30 minutes
Preheat broiler to 400 F and mix the lemon juice, garlic, salt, pepper, and oil in a bowl. Brush the pork with the mixture, place in a baking sheet, and cook for 6 minutes on each side until browned. Share into 6 plates. Melt butter in a small wok or pan and cook broccoli tips for 5 minutes until tender. Drizzle with white wine, sprinkle with salt and pepper and cook for another 5 minutes. Ladle broccoli to the side of the chops and serve with hot sauce.
Per serving: Cal 549, Net Carbs 2g, Fat 48g, Protein 26g

Jerk Pork Pot Roast

Ingredients for 8 servings
4-pound pork roast
1 tbsp olive oil
¼ cup Jerk spice blend
½ cup beef stock

Directions and Total Time: approx. 4 hours 20 minutes
Rub the pork with olive oil and the spice blend. Heat a dutch oven over medium heat and sear the meat well on all sides. Add the beef broth. Cover the pot, reduce the heat, and let cook for 4 hours.
Per serving: Cal 282; Net Carbs 0g; Fat 24g; Protein 23g

Swiss Pork Patties with Salad

Ingredients for 4 servings
1 lb ground pork
3 tbsp olive oil
2 hearts romaine lettuce, torn
2 firm tomatoes, sliced
¼ red onion, sliced
3 oz Swiss cheese, shredded

Directions and Total Time: approx. 30 minutes
Season pork with salt and pepper, mix, and shape several medium-sized patties. Heat 2 tbsp oil in a skillet and fry the patties on both sides for 10 minutes. Transfer to a wire rack to drain oil. When cooled, cut into quarters. Mix lettuce, tomatoes, and onion in a bowl, season with oil, salt and pepper. Toss and add the patties on top. Microwave the cheese for 90 seconds, drizzle it over the salad.
Per serving: Cal 310, Net Carbs 2g, Fat 23g, Protein 22g

Maple Scallion Pork Bites

Ingredients for 4 servings
½ cup + 1 tbsp red wine
1 tbsp + 1/3 cup tamari sauce
1 pork tenderloin, cubed
½ cup sugar-free maple syrup
½ cup sesame seeds
1 tbsp sesame oil
1 tsp freshly pureed garlic
½ tsp freshly grated ginger
1 scallion, finely chopped

Directions and Total Time: approx. 50 minutes
Preheat oven to 350 F. In a zipper bag, combine ½ cup of red wine with 1 tbsp of tamari sauce. Add in pork cubes, seal the bag, and marinate the meat in the fridge overnight. Remove from the fridge and drain. Pour maple syrup and sesame seeds into two separate bowls; roll the pork in maple syrup and then in the sesame seeds. Place on a greased baking sheet and bake for 35 minutes. In a bowl, mix the remaining wine, tamari sauce, sesame oil, garlic, and ginger. Pour the sauce into a bowl. Transfer pork to a platter and garnish with scallions. Serve with sauce.
Per serving: Cal 352; Net Carbs 6.4g; Fat 18g; Protein 39g

Pork Medallions with Pancetta

Ingredients for 4 servings
1 lb pork loin, cut into medallions
2 onions, chopped
6 pancetta slices, chopped
½ cup vegetable stock
Salt and black pepper, to taste

Directions and Total Time: approx. 55 minutes
Set a pan over medium heat, and cook the pancetta until crispy; remove to a plate. Add onions and stir-fry for 5 minutes; set aside to the same plate as pancetta. Add pork medallions to the pan, season with pepper and salt, brown for 3 minutes on each side, turn, reduce heat, and cook for 7 minutes. Stir in the stock, and cook for 2 minutes. Return the pancetta and onions and cook for 1 minute.

Per serving: Cal 325, Net Carbs 6g, Fat 18g, Protein 36g

Golden Pork Chops with Mushrooms

Ingredients for 6 servings
2 (14-oz) cans Mushroom soup
1 onion, chopped
6 pork chops
½ cup sliced mushrooms
Salt and black pepper to taste

Directions and Total Time: approx. 1 hour 15 minutes
Preheat the oven to 375 F. Season the pork chops with salt and pepper, and place them in a baking dish. Combine the soup, mushrooms, and onions in a bowl. Pour this mixture over the pork chops. Bake for 45 minutes.

Per serving: Cal 403; Net Carbs 8g; Fat 32.6g; Protein 19g

Cumin Pork Chops

Ingredients for 4 servings
4 pork chops
¾ cup cumin powder
1 tsp chili powder
Salt and black pepper to taste

Directions and Total Time: approx. 25 minutes
In a bowl, combine the cumin with black pepper, salt, and chili. Place in the pork chops and rub them well. Heat a grill over medium temperature, add in the pork chops, cook for 5 minutes, flip, and cook for 5 minutes.

Per serving: Cal 349; Net Carbs 4g; Fat 18.6g; Protein 42g

SEAFOOD

Wine Shrimp Scampi Pizza

Ingredients for 4 servings
½ cup almond flour
¼ tsp salt
2 tbsp ground psyllium husk
3 tbsp olive oil
2 tbsp butter
2 garlic cloves, minced
¼ cup white wine
½ tsp dried basil
½ tsp dried parsley
½ lemon, juiced
½ lb shrimp, deveined
2 cups grated cheese blend
½ tsp Italian seasoning
¼ cup grated Parmesan

Directions and Total Time: approx. 35 minutes
Preheat oven to 390 F and line a baking sheet with parchment paper. In a bowl, mix almond flour, salt, psyllium powder, 1 tbsp of olive oil, and 1 cup of lukewarm water until dough forms. Spread the mixture on the pizza pan and bake for 10 minutes. Heat butter and the remaining olive oil in a skillet. Sauté garlic for 30 seconds. Mix in white wine, reduce by half, and stir in basil, parsley and lemon juice. Stir in shrimp and cook for 3 minutes. Mix in the cheese blend and Italian seasoning. Let the cheese melt, 3 minutes. Spread the shrimp mixture on the crust and top with Parmesan cheese. Bake for 5 minutes or until Parmesan melts. Slice and serve warm.
Per serving: Cal 423; Net Carbs 3.9g; Fats 34g; Protein 23g

Shallot Mussel with Shirataki

Ingredients for 4 servings
2 (8 oz) packs angel hair shirataki
1 lb mussels
1 cup white wine
4 tbsp olive oil
3 shallots, finely chopped
6 garlic cloves, minced
2 tsp red chili flakes
½ cup fish stock
1 ½ cups heavy cream
2 tbsp chopped fresh parsley
Salt and black pepper to taste

Directions and Total Time: approx. 25 minutes
Bring 2 cups of water to a boil in a pot. Strain the shirataki pasta and rinse well under hot running water. Drain and transfer to the boiling water. Cook for 3 minutes and strain again. Place a large dry skillet and stir-fry the shirataki pasta until visibly dry, 1-2 minutes; set aside. Pour mussels and white wine into a pot, cover, and cook for 3-4 minutes. Strain mussels and reserve the cooking liquid. Let cool, discard any closed mussels, and remove the meat out of ¾ of the mussel shells. Set aside with the remaining mussels in the shells. Heat olive oil in a skillet and sauté shallots, garlic, and chili flakes for 3 minutes. Mix in reduced wine and fish stock. Allow boiling and whisk in remaining butter and then the heavy cream. Season with salt, and pepper, and mix in parsley. Pour in shirataki pasta, mussels and toss well in the sauce. Serve.
Per serving: Cal 471; Net Carbs 6.9g; Fats 34g; Protein 18g

Nori Shrimp Rolls

Ingredients for 5 servings
2 cups cooked shrimp
1 tbsp Sriracha sauce
¼ cucumber, julienned
5 hand roll nori sheets
¼ cup mayonnaise
1 tbsp dill

Directions and Total Time: approx. 10 minutes
Chop the shrimp and combine with mayo, dill, and sriracha sauce in a bowl. Place a single nori sheet on a flat surface and spread about a fifth of the shrimp mixture. Roll the nori sheet as desired. Repeat with the other ingredients.
Per serving: Cal 130; Net Carbs 1g; Fat 10g; Protein 8.7g

Hazelnut-Crusted Salmon

Ingredients for 4 servings
4 salmon fillets
Salt and black pepper to taste
¼ cup mayonnaise
½ cup chopped hazelnuts
1 chopped shallot
2 tsp lemon zest
1 tbsp olive oil
1 cup heavy cream

Directions and Total Time: approx. 35 minutes
Preheat oven to 360 F. Brush the salmon with mayonnaise and coat with hazelnuts. Place in a lined baking dish and bake for 15 minutes. Heat olive oil in a saucepan and sauté shallot for 3 minutes. Stir in lemon zest and heavy cream and bring to a boil; cook until thickened, 5 minutes. Adjust seasoning and drizzle the sauce over the fish to serve.
Per serving: Cal 563; Net Carbs 6g; Fat 47g; Protein 34g

Fish & Cauliflower Parmesan Gratin

Ingredients for 4 servings
1 head cauliflower, cut into florets
2 cod fillets, cubed
3 white fish fillets, cubed
1 tbsp butter, melted
1 cup crème fraiche
¼ cup grated Parmesan
Grated Parmesan for topping

Directions and Total Time: approx. 40 minutes
Preheat oven to 400 F. Coat fish cubes and broccoli with butter. Spread in a greased baking dish. Mix crème fraiche with Parmesan cheese, pour and smear the cream on the fish, and sprinkle with some more Parmesan cheese. Bake for 25-30 minutes. Let sit for 5 minutes and serve in plates.
Per serving: Cal 354; Net Carbs 4g; Fat 17g; Protein 28g

Broccoli & Fish Gratin

Ingredients for 4 servings
¼ cup grated Pecorino Romano cheese + some more
2 salmon fillets, cubed
3 white fish, cubed
1 broccoli, cut into florets
1 tbsp butter, melted
Salt and black pepper to taste
1 cup crème fraiche

Directions and Total Time: approx. 45 minutes
Preheat oven to 400 F. Toss the fish cubes and broccoli in butter and season with salt and pepper. Spread in a greased dish. Mix crème fraiche with Pecorino Romano cheese, pour and smear the cream on the fish. Bake for 30 minutes. Serve with lemon-mustard asparagus.
Per serving: Cal 354; Net Carbs 4g; Fat 17g; Protein 28g

Salmon Caesar Salad with Poached Eggs

Ingredients for 4 servings
½ cup chopped smoked salmon
2 tbsp heinz low carb caesar dressing
3 cups water
8 eggs
2 cups torn romaine lettuce
6 slices pancetta

Directions and Total Time: approx. 15 minutes
Boil water in a pot for 5 minutes. Crack each egg into a small bowl and gently slide into the water. Poach for 2-3 minutes, remove, and transfer to a paper towel to dry. Poach the remaining 7 eggs. Put the pancetta in a skillet and fry for 6 minutes, turning once. Allow cooling, and chop into small pieces. Toss the lettuce, smoked salmon, pancetta, and caesar dressing in a salad bowl. Top with two eggs each, and serve immediately.
Per serving: Cal 260; Net Carbs 5g; Fat 21g; Protein 8g

Avocado & Cauliflower Salad with Prawns

Ingredients for 6 servings
1 cauliflower head, florets only
1 lb medium-sized prawns
¼ cup + 1 tbsp olive oil
1 avocado, chopped
3 tbsp chopped dill
¼ cup lemon juice
2 tbsp lemon zest

Directions and Total Time: approx. 30 minutes
Heat 1 tbsp olive oil in a skillet and cook the prawns for 8-10 minutes. Microwave cauliflower for 5 minutes. Place prawns, cauliflower, and avocado in a large bowl. Whisk together the remaining olive oil, lemon zest, juice, dill, and some salt and pepper, in another bowl. Pour the dressing over, toss to combine and serve immediately.
Per serving: Cal 214; Net Carbs 5g; Fat 17g; Protein 15g

Fish Fritters

Ingredients for 4 servings
1 pound cod fillets, sliced
¼ cup mayonnaise
¼ cup almond flour
2 eggs
Salt and black pepper to taste
1 cup Swiss cheese, grated
1 tbsp chopped dill
3 tbsp olive oil

Directions and Total Time: approx. 40 min + cooling time
Mix the fish, mayo, flour, eggs, salt, pepper, Swiss cheese, and dill, in a bowl. Cover the bowl with plastic wrap and refrigerate for 2 hours. Warm olive oil and fetch 2 tbsp of fish mixture into the skillet, use the back of a spatula to flatten the top. Cook for 4 minutes, flip, and fry for 4 more. Remove onto a wire rack and repeat until the fish batter is over; add more oil if needed.
Per serving: Cal 633; Net Carbs 7g; Fat 46.9g; Protein 39g

VEGAN & VEGETARIAN

Mint Ice Cream

Ingredients for 4 servings
2 avocados, pitted
1 ¼ cups coconut cream
½ tsp vanilla extract
2 tbsp erythritol
2 tsp chopped mint leaves

Directions and Total Time: approx. 10 min+ chilling time
Into a blender, spoon avocado pulps, pour in coconut cream, vanilla extract, erythritol, and mint leaves. Process until smooth. Pour the mixture into your ice cream maker and freeze according to the manufacturer's instructions. When ready, remove and scoop the ice cream into bowls.
Per serving: Cal 370; Net Carbs 4g; Fat 38g; Protein 4g

Eggplant & Goat Cheese Pizza

Ingredients for 4 servings
4 tbsp olive oil
2 eggplants, sliced lengthwise
1 cup tomato sauce
2 garlic cloves, minced
1 red onion, sliced
12 oz goat cheese, crumbled
Salt and black pepper to taste
½ tsp cinnamon powder
1 cup mozzarella, shredded
2 tbsp oregano, chopped

Directions and Total Time: approx. 45 minutes
Line a baking sheet with parchment paper. Lay the eggplant slices in a baking dish and drizzle with some olive oil. Bake for 20 minutes at 390 F. Heat the remaining olive oil in a skillet and sauté garlic and onion for 3 minutes. Stir in goat cheese and tomato sauce and season with salt and pepper. Simmer for 10 minutes. Remove eggplant from the oven and spread the cheese sauce on top. Sprinkle with mozzarella cheese and oregano. Bake further for 10 minutes until the cheese melts. Slice to serve.
Per serving: Cal 557; Net Carbs 8.3g; Fat 44g; Protein 33.7g

Charred Asparagus with Creamy Sauce

Ingredients for 4 servings
½ lb asparagus, no hard stalks
Salt and chili pepper to taste
4 tbsp flax seed powder
½ cup coconut cream
1 cup butter, melted
⅓ cup mozzarella, grated
2 tbsp olive oil
Juice of half lemon

Directions and Total Time: approx. 12 minutes
Heat olive oil in a saucepan and roast the asparagus until lightly charred. Season with salt and pepper; set aside. Melt half of butter in a pan until nutty and golden brown. Stir in lemon juice and pour the mixture over the asparagus. In a safe microwave bowl, mix flax seed powder with ½ cup water and let sit for 5 minutes. Microwave flax egg 1-2 minutes, then pour into a blender. Add the remaining butter, mozzarella cheese, coconut cream, salt, and chili pepper. Puree until well combined and smooth. Serve.

Per serving: Cal 442; Net Carbs 5.4g; Fat 45g; Protein 5.9g

Tomato & Mozzarella Caprese Bake

Ingredients for 4 servings
4 tbsp olive oil
4 tomatoes, sliced
1 cup fresh mozzarella, sliced
2 tbsp basil pesto
1 cup mayonnaise
2 oz Parmesan cheese, grated

Directions and Total Time: approx. 25 minutes
In a baking dish, arrange tomatoes and mozzarella slices. In a bowl, mix pesto, mayonnaise, 1 oz of Parmesan cheese, salt, and pepper; mix to combine. Spread this mixture over tomatoes and mozzarella cheese, and top with remaining Parmesan cheese. Bake for 20 minutes at 360 F. Remove, allow cooling slightly, and slice to serve.

Per serving: Cal 420; Net Carbs 4.9g; Fat 36.6g; Protein 17g

Sweet Onion & Goat Cheese Pizza

Ingredients for 4 servings
2 cups grated mozzarella
2 tbsp cream cheese, softened
2 large eggs, beaten
⅓ cup almond flour
1 tsp dried Italian seasoning
2 tbsp butter
2 red onions, thinly sliced
1 cup crumbled goat cheese
1 tbs almond milk
1 cup curly endive, chopped

Directions and Total Time: approx. 35 minutes
Preheat oven to 390 F and line a round pizza pan with parchment paper. Microwave the mozzarella and cream cheeses for 1 minute. Remove and mix in eggs, almond flour, and Italian seasoning. Spread the dough on the pizza pan and bake for 6 minutes. Melt butter in a skillet and stir in onions, salt, and pepper and cook on low heat with frequent stirring until caramelized, 15-20 minutes. In a bowl, mix goat cheese with almond milk and spread on the crust. Top with the caramelized onions. Bake for 10 minutes. Scatter curly endive on top, slice and serve.
Per serving: Cal 317; Net Carbs 3.1g; Fats 20g; Protein 28g

Vegan BBQ Tofu Kabobs with Green Dip

Ingredients for 4 servings
½ tbsp BBQ sauce
1 lb extra firm tofu, cubed
1 tbsp vegan butter, melted
1 cup canola oil
5 tbsp fresh cilantro, chopped
3 tbsp fresh basil, chopped
2 garlic cloves
Juice of ½ a lime
4 tbsp capers
Salt and black pepper to taste

Directions and Total Time: approx. 20 minutes
In a blender, add cilantro, basil, garlic, lemon juice, capers, 2/3 cup of canola oil, salt and pepper. Process until smooth. Set aside. Thread the tofu cubes on wooden skewers to fit into your grill pan. Season with salt and brush with the BBQ sauce. Brush the grill pan with remaining canola oil and cook the tofu until browned on both sides. Serve.
Per serving: Cal 471; Net Carbs 3.8g; Fat 47g; Protein 11.9g

One-Pot Spicy Brussel Sprouts with Carrots

Ingredients for 4 servings
1 pound Brussels sprouts
¼ cup olive oil
4 green onions, chopped
1 carrot, grated
Salt and black pepper to taste
Hot chili sauce

Directions and Total Time: approx. 15 minutes
Sauté green onions in warm olive oil for 2 minutes. Stir in salt and pepper; transfer to a plate. Trim the Brussel sprouts and cut in halves. Leave the small ones as wholes. Pour the Brussel sprouts with and carrot into the same saucepan and stir-fry until softened but al dente. Season with salt and pepper, stir in onions, and heat for a few seconds. Top with the hot chili sauce. Serve.

Per serving: Cal 198; Net Carbs 6.5g; Fat 14g; Protein 4.9g

Tofu Nuggets with Cilantro Dip

Ingredients for 4 servings
1 lime, ½ juiced and ½ cut into wedges
1 ½ cups olive oil
28 oz tofu, pressed and cubed
1 egg, lightly beaten
1 cup golden flaxseed meal
1 ripe avocado, chopped
½ tbsp chopped cilantro
Salt and black pepper to taste
½ tbsp olive oil

Directions and Total Time: approx. 25 minutes
Heat olive oil in a deep skillet. Coat tofu cubes in the egg and then in the flaxseed meal. Fry until golden brown. Transfer to a plate. Place avocado, cilantro, salt, pepper, and lime juice in a blender; puree until smooth. Spoon into a bowl, add tofu nuggets, and lime wedges to serve.

Per serving: Cal 665; Net Carbs 6.2g, Fat 54g, Protein 32g

Zucchini-Cranberry Cake Squares

Ingredients for 6 servings
1 ¼ cups chopped zucchinis
2 tbsp olive oil
½ cup dried cranberries
1 lemon, zested
3 eggs
1 ½ cups almond flour
½ tsp baking powder
1 tsp cinnamon powder
A pinch of salt

Directions and Total Time: approx. 45 minutes
Preheat oven to 350 F and line a square cake tin with parchment paper. Combine zucchinis, olive oil, cranberries, lemon zest, and eggs in a bowl until evenly combined. Sift flour, baking powder, and cinnamon powder into the mixture and fold with the salt. Pour the mixture into the cake tin and bake for 30 minutes. Remove; allow cooling in the tin for 10 minutes and transfer the cake to a wire rack to cool completely. Cut into squares and serve.
Per serving: Cal 121; Net Carbs 2.5g, Fat 10g, Protein 4g

Egg Cauli Fried Rice with Grilled Cheese

Ingredients for 4 servings
2 cups cauliflower rice, steamed
½ lb halloumi, cut into ¼ to ½ inch slabs
1 tbsp ghee
4 eggs, beaten
1 green bell pepper, chopped
¼ cup green beans, chopped
1 tsp soy sauce
2 tbsp chopped parsley

Directions and Total Time: approx. 10 minutes
Melt ghee in a skillet and pour in the eggs. Swirl the pan to spread the eggs around and cook for 1 minute. Move the scrambled eggs to the side of the skillet, add bell pepper and green beans, and sauté for 3 minutes. Pour in the cauli rice and cook for 2 minutes. Top with soy sauce; combine evenly, and cook for 2 minutes. Dish into plates, garnish with the parsley, and set aside. Preheat a grill pan and grill halloumi cheese on both sides until the cheese lightly browns. Place on the side of the rice and serve warm.
Per serving: Cal 275; Net Carbs 4.5g, Fat 19g, Protein 15g

Strawberry Faux Oats

Ingredients for 2 servings
2 tbsp coconut flour
2 tbsp golden flaxseed meal
2 tbsp chia seeds
2 tbsp heavy cream
½ cup almond milk
3 tbsp sugar-free maple syrup
1 tsp vanilla extract
1 cup strawberries, halved
¼ cup desiccated coconut

Directions and Total Time: approx. 20 minutes
Combine coconut flour, flaxseed meal, and chia seeds in a saucepan. Stir in heavy cream, almond milk, maple syrup, and vanilla extract. Place the pan over medium heat, whisk the Ingredients for 10 minutes. Pour the mixture into 2 serving bowls and top with strawberries and desiccated coconut. Drizzle with some more maple syrup and serve.
Per serving: Cal 289; Net Carbs 6g, Fat 18.5g, Protein 5g

Cheese Quesadillas with Fruit Salad

Ingredients for 2 servings
2 large zero carb tortillas
1 cup grated cheddar cheese
2 green onions, chopped
1 cup mixed berries
½ tsp cinnamon powder
½ lemon, juiced
1 cup Greek yogurt
Sugar-free maple syrup to taste

Directions and Total Time: approx. 10 minutes
Divide the tortillas into two, top half each with the cheddar cheese and spring onions, and cover with the halves. Place in a skillet and heat until golden and the cheese melted. Remove onto a plate, allow cooling, and cut into four wedges. Combine berries, cinnamon powder, lemon juice, Greek yogurt, and maple syrup in a bowl. Divide into 2 bowls and serve with the quesadillas.
Per serving: Cal 135; Net Carbs 3g, Fat 13.5g, Protein 3.5g

Mushroom & Broccoli Pizza

Ingredients for 4 servings
½ cup almond flour
¼ tsp salt
2 tbsp ground psyllium husk
2 tbsp olive oil
1 cup sliced fresh mushrooms
1 white onion, thinly sliced
3 cups broccoli florets
4 garlic cloves, minced
½ cup sugar-free pizza sauce
4 tomatoes, sliced
1 ½ cups grated mozzarella
⅓ cup grated Parmesan

Directions and Total Time: approx. 25 minutes
Preheat oven to 390 F and line a baking sheet with parchment paper. In a bowl, mix almond flour, salt, psyllium powder, 1 tbsp of olive oil, and 1 cup of lukewarm water until dough forms. Spread the mixture on the pizza pan and bake for 10 minutes. Heat the remaining olive oil in a skillet and sauté mushrooms, onion, garlic, and broccoli for 5 minutes. Spread the pizza sauce on the crust and top with the broccoli mixture, tomato, and mozzarella and Parmesan cheeses. Bake for 5 minutes. Serve sliced.
Per serving: Cal 180; Net Carbs 3.6g; Fats 9.4g; Protein 17g

Tofu Radish Bowls

Ingredients for 4 servings
¼ cup chopped baby bella mushrooms
2 yellow bell peppers, chopped
1 (14 oz) block tofu, cubed
1 tbsp + 1 tbsp olive oil
1 ½ cups shredded radishes
½ cup chopped white onions
4 eggs
1/3 cup tomato salsa
A handful chopped parsley
1 avocado, and chopped

Directions and Total Time: approx. 35 minutes
Heat 1 tbsp olive oil in a skillet and add the tofu, radishes, onions, mushrooms, and bell peppers. Season with salt and pepper; cook for 10 minutes. Share into 4 bowls. Heat the remaining oil in the skillet, crack an egg into the pan, and cook until the white sets, but the yolk quite runny. Transfer to the top of one tofu-radish hash bowl and make the remaining eggs. Top the bowls with tomato salsa, parsley, and avocado. Serve.
Per serving: Cal 353; Net Carbs 5.9g, Fat 25g, Protein 19g

Mascarpone and Kale Asian Casserole

Ingredients for 4 servings
2 cups tofu, grilled and cubed
1 cup smoked seitan, chopped
1 cup mascarpone cheese
1 tbsp mustard powder
1 tbsp plain vinegar
1 ¼ cups cheddar, shredded
½ cup kale, chopped
2 tbsp olive oil

Directions and Total Time: approx. 30 minutes
Mix the mascarpone cheese, mustard powder, plain vinegar, kale, and cheddar cheese in a greased baking dish. Top with the tofu, seitan, and season with salt and black pepper. Bake in the oven until the casserole is golden brown on top, for about 15 to 20 minutes, at 400 F. Serve.
Per serving: Cal 612; Net Carbs 9.1g; Fat 51g; Protein 30.5g

Cauliflower Couscous & Halloumi Packets

Ingredients for 4 servings
2 heads cauliflower, chopped
¼ cup vegetable broth
1 lemon, juiced
2 tbsp sugar-free maple syrup
1 red bell pepper, chopped
1 orange bell pepper, chopped
¼ cup cubed halloumi
Olive oil to drizzle

Directions and Total Time: approx. 25 minutes
Preheat oven to 350 F. Put cauliflower in a food processor and pulse until a coarse consistency is achieved. Pour the couscous and vegetable stock into a pot and cook for 2-3 minutes. Drain and set aside. In a bowl, whisk lemon juice and maple syrup, and set aside. Cut out two 2 x 15 inches parchment papers onto a flat surface spoon the couscous in the middle of each, top with bell peppers, halloumi cheese, and drizzle the dressing on top. Wrap papers into parcels and place on a baking tray; cook for 15 minutes. Remove and carefully open the pouches. Serve warm.
Per serving: Cal 240; Net Carbs 4.7g, Fat 19g, Protein 5.1g

Mushroom White Pizza

Ingredients for 4 servings
2 tbsp flax egg + 6 tbsp water
½ cup mayonnaise
¾ cup almond flour
1 tbsp psyllium husk powder
1 tsp baking soda
½ tsp salt
¼ cup mushrooms, sliced
1 tbsp oregano
1 tbsp basil pesto
2 tbsp olive oil
Salt and black pepper
½ cup coconut cream
¾ cup Parmesan, shredded
6 black olives

Directions and Total Time: approx. 35 minutes
Combine the flax seed powder with water and allow sitting to thicken for 5 minutes. Whisk in mayonnaise, almond flour, psyllium husk powder, baking soda, and salt. Allow sitting for 5 minutes. Pour the batter into a greased baking sheet. Bake for 10 minutes at 350 F. In a bowl, mix mushrooms with pesto, olive oil, salt, and pepper. Remove the crust from the oven and spread the coconut cream on top. Add the mushroom mixture and Parmesan cheese. Bake the pizza further until the cheese melts, for 10 minutes. Spread the olives on top and serve.
Per serving: Cal 346; Net Carbs 5.5g; Fat 32.7g; Protein 8g

Garam Masala Traybake

Ingredients for 4 servings
3 tbsp butter
3 cups tempeh slices
1 turnip, sliced
Salt to taste
2 tbsp garam masala
1 cup mushrooms, sliced
1 ¼ cups coconut cream
1 tbsp fresh cilantro, chopped

Directions and Total Time: approx. 30 minutes
Place a skillet and melt butter. Fry tempeh for 4 minutes. Stir half of the garam masala into the tempeh until evenly mixed and turn the heat off. Transfer the tempeh with the spice into a baking dish and set aside. In a bowl, mix the mushrooms, turnip, coconut cream, cilantro, and remaining garam masala. Pour the mixture over tempeh and bake for 20 minutes at 400 F. Garnish with cilantro.
Per serving: Cal 591; Net Carbs 9.4g; Fat 48.4g; Protein 28g

Walnut Chocolate Squares

Ingredients for 6 servings
3½ oz dairy-free dark chocolate
4 tbsp vegan butter
1 pinch salt
¼ cup walnut butter
½ tsp vanilla extract
¼ cup chopped walnuts

Directions and Total Time: approx. 10 minutes
Microwave chocolate and vegan butter for 2 minutes. Remove and mix in salt, walnut butter, and vanilla extract. Grease a small baking sheet with cooking spray and line with parchment paper. Pour in the batter and top with walnuts and chill in the refrigerator. Cut into squares.
Per serving: Cal 125; Net Carbs 3g; Fat 10g; Protein 2g

Cauliflower & Broccoli Gratin with Seitan

Ingredients for 4 servings
4 tbsp avocado oil
2 shallots, chopped
2 cups broccoli florets
1 cup cauliflower florets
2 cups seitan, crumbled
1 cup heavy cream
2 tbsp mustard powder
5 oz Pecorino, shredded
4 tbsp rosemary, chopped
Salt and black pepper to taste

Directions and Total Time: approx. 40 minutes
Heat half of the avocado oil in a pot and add shallots, broccoli, and cauliflower and cook for 6 minutes. Transfer the vegetables to a baking dish. Warm the remaining avocado oil in a skillet and cook the seitan until browned. Mix heavy cream and mustard powder in a bowl. Then, pour the mixture over the vegetables. Scatter seitan and Pecorino cheese on top and sprinkle with rosemary, salt ,and pepper. Bake for 15 minutes at 400 F. Serve.
Per serving: Cal 753; Net Carbs 12g; Fat 37g; Protein 86g

Baked Creamy Brussels Sprouts

Ingredients for 4 servings
3 tbsp ghee
1 cup tempeh, cubed
1 lb Brussels sprouts, halved
5 garlic cloves, minced
1 ¼ cups crème fraîche
1 ⅓ cups cheddar, shredded
¼ cup Gruyère, shredded
Salt and black pepper to taste

Directions and Total Time: approx. 25 minutes
Melt ghee in a large skillet and fry tempeh for 6 minutes; set aside. Pour Brussels sprouts and garlic into the skillet and sauté until nice color forms. Stir in crème fraîche and simmer for 4 minutes. Add tempeh cubes and mix well. Pour the sautéed ingredients into a baking dish, sprinkle with cheddar cheese and Gruyère cheese. Bake for 10 minutes at 400 F or until golden brown on top. Serve.
Per serving: Cal 563; Net Carbs 8.7g; Fat 44g; Protein 25.2g

Mom's Cheesy Pizza

Ingredients for 4 servings
1 cup sliced mozzarella
1 cup grated mozzarella
3 tbsp grated Parmesan
½ cup almond flour
¼ tsp salt
2 tbsp ground psyllium husk
1 tbsp olive oil
½ cup sugar-free pizza sauce
2 tsp Italian seasoning
1 cup lukewarm water

Directions and Total Time: approx. 35 minutes
Preheat oven to 390 F and line a pizza pan with parchment paper. In a bowl, mix almond flour, salt, psyllium powder, olive oil, and water until dough forms. Spread the mixture on the pizza pan and bake for 10 minutes. Remove the crust and spread the pizza sauce on top. Add the sliced mozzarella, grated mozzarella, Parmesan cheese, and Italian seasoning. Bake for 18 minutes. Slice and serve.
Per serving: Cal 193; Net Carbs 3.2g; Fats 10g; Protein 19g

Key Lime Truffles

Ingredients for 6 servings
¼ cup cocoa powder mixed with 2 tbsp swerve sugar
1 cup dark chocolate, chopped
2/3 cup heavy cream
2 tsp lime extract

Directions and Total Time: approx. 5 min + cooling time
Heat heavy cream in a pan over low heat until tiny bubbles form around the edges of the pan. Turn the heat off. Pour dark chocolate into the pan, swirl the pan to allow the hot cream to spread over the chocolate, and then gently stir the mixture until smooth. Mix in lime extract and transfer to a bowl. Refrigerate for 4 hours. Line 2 baking trays with parchment papers; set one aside and pour cocoa powder mixture onto the other. Take out the chocolate mixture; form bite-size balls out of the mix and roll all round in the cocoa powder to completely coat. Place the truffles on the baking tray and refrigerate for 30 minutes before serving.
Per serving: Cal 143; Net Carbs 0.6g, Fat 12g, Protein 2.4g

Lemon Sponge Cake with Cream

Ingredients for 4 servings
1 tbsp swerve confectioner's sugar, for dusting
4 large lemons, chopped
¼ cup sugar-free maple syrup
½ cup butter, softened
½ cup erythritol
1 tsp vanilla extract
½ cup almond flour, sifted
3 large eggs, lightly beaten
½ cup heavy cream

Directions and Total Time: approx. 40 minutes
Place the chopped lemons in a saucepan. Add in sugar-free maple syrup and simmer over low heat for 30 minutes. Pour the mixture into a blender and process until smooth. Pour into a jar and set aside. Preheat oven to 350 F, grease two (8-inch) springform pans with cooking spray, and line with parchment paper. In a bowl, cream the butter, erythritol, and vanilla extract with an electric whisk until light and fluffy. Pour in the eggs gradually while beating until fully mixed. Carefully fold in the almond flour and share the mixture into the cake pans. Bake for 30 minutes or until springy when touched and a toothpick inserted comes out clean. Remove and let cool for 5 minutes before turning out onto a wire rack. In a bowl, whip heavy cream until a soft peak forms. Spoon onto the bottom sides of the cake and spread the lemon puree on top. Sandwich both cakes and sift confectioner's sugar on top. Slice and serve.
Per serving: Cal 266; Net Carbs 4.6g; Fat 25g; Protein 6g

Zucchini Cake Slices

Ingredients for 4 servings
1 cup butter, softened
1 cup erythritol
4 eggs
2/3 cup coconut flour
2 tsp baking powder
2/3 cup ground almonds
1 lemon, zested and juiced
1 cup finely grated zucchini
1 cup crème fraiche
1 tbsp chopped walnuts

Directions and Total Time: approx. 30 min + cooling time
Preheat oven to 375 F, grease a springform pan with and line with parchment paper. In a bowl, beat butter and erythritol until creamy and pale. Add eggs one after another while whisking. Sift coconut flour and baking powder into the mixture and stir along with ground almonds, lemon zest, juice, and zucchini. Spoon the mixture into the pan and bake for 40 minutes or until risen and a toothpick inserted into the cake comes out clean. Let cool inside the pan for 10 minutes, and transfer to a wire rack. Spread crème fraiche on top and sprinkle with walnuts to serve.
Per serving: Cal 778; Net Carbs 3.7g, Fat 71g, Protein 32g

Blackberry Lemon Tarte Tatin

Ingredients for 4 servings
¼ cup butter, cold and crumbled
¼ cup almond flour
3 tbsp coconut flour
½ tsp salt
3 tbsp erythritol
1 ½ tsp vanilla extract
4 whole eggs
4 tbsp melted butter
3 tsp swerve brown sugar
1 cup fresh blackberries
1 tsp vanilla extract
1 lemon, juiced
1 cup ricotta cheese
4 fresh basil leaves to garnish
1 egg, lightly beaten

Directions and Total Time: approx. 50 minutes
Preheat oven to 350 F. In a bowl, mix almond and coconut flour, and salt. Add in butter and mix until crumbly. Mix in erythritol and vanilla extract. Pour in the 4 eggs and mix until formed into a ball. Flatten the dough on a clean flat surface, cover in plastic wrap, and refrigerate for 1 hour. Dust a clean flat surface with almond flour, unwrap the dough, and roll out the dough into a circle. In a greased baking pan, mix butter, swerve brown sugar, blackberries, vanilla extract, and lemon juice. Arrange blackberries uniformly across the pan. Lay the pastry over the fruit filling and tuck the sides into the pan. Brush with beaten egg and bake for 40 minutes. Turn the pie onto a plate, crumble ricotta cheese on top, and garnish with basil.
Per serving: Cal 465; Net Carbs 5.8g, Fat 41g, Protein 16g

Avocado Truffles with Chocolate Coating

Ingredients for 6 servings
1 ripe avocado, pitted
½ tsp vanilla extract
½ tsp lemon zest
5 oz dark chocolate
1 tbsp coconut oil
1 tbsp cocoa powder

Directions and Total Time: approx. 5 minutes
Scoop pulp of the avocado into a bowl and mix with vanilla using an immersion blender. Stir in lemon zest and a pinch of salt. Microwave chocolate and coconut oil for 1 minute. Add to the avocado mixture and stir. Allow cooling to firm up a bit. Form balls out of the mix. Roll each ball in the cocoa powder and serve immediately.
Per serving: Cal 70; Net Carbs 2g; Fat 6g; Protein 2g

Strawberry Blackberry Pie

Ingredients for 4 servings
¼ cup butter, cold and crumbled
2 ¼ cup strawberries and blackberries
1 vanilla pod, bean paste extracted
¼ cup almond flour
3 tbsp coconut flour
½ tsp salt
3 tbsp + 1 cup erythritol
1 ½ tsp vanilla extract
4 whole eggs
1 egg, beaten

Directions and Total Time: approx. 30 min + cooling time
Preheat oven to 350 F. In a bowl, mix almond and coconut flours, and salt. Add in butter and mix until crumbly. Stir in 3 tbsp of erythritol and vanilla extract. Pour in the 4 eggs one after another while mixing until formed into a ball. Cover the dough with plastic wrap, and refrigerate for 1 hour. Dust a clean flat surface with almond flour, unwrap the dough, and roll out into a large rectangle to fit into a greased pie pan; prick the base of the crust. Bake until golden. In a bowl, mix berries, remaining erythritol, and vanilla paste. Spoon mixture into the pie and use the pastry strips to create a lattice over the berries. Brush with beaten egg and bake for 30 minutes. Slice and serve.
Per serving: Cal 262; Net Carbs 3g, Fat 21.7g, Protein 9g

Berry Hazelnut Trifle

Ingredients for 4 servings
1 ½ ripe avocados
¾ cup coconut cream
Zest and juice of ½ a lemon
1 tbsp vanilla extract
3 oz fresh strawberries
2 oz toasted hazelnuts

Directions and Total Time: approx. 5 minutes
In a bowl, add avocado pulp, coconut cream, lemon zest and juice, and half of the vanilla extract. Mix with an immersion blender. Put the strawberries and remaining vanilla in another bowl and use a fork to mash the fruits. In a tall glass, alternate layering the cream and strawberry mixtures. Drop a few hazelnuts on each and serve.
Per serving: Cal 360; Net Carbs 7g; Fat 34g; Protein 4g

Coconut Chocolate Fudge

Ingredients for 6 servings
2 cups coconut cream
1 tsp vanilla extract
3 oz vegan butter
3 oz dark chocolate, chopped
Swerve sugar for sprinkling

Directions and Total Time: approx. 20 min+ chilling time
Pour coconut cream and vanilla into a saucepan and bring to a boil over medium heat, then simmer until reduced by half, about 15 minutes. Stir in vegan butter until the batter is smooth. Add in dark chocolate and stir until melted. Pour the mixture into a baking sheet; chill in the fridge. Cut into squares, sprinkle with swerve sugar, and serve.
Per serving: Cal 116; Net Carbs 3g; Fat 11g; Protein 2g

Raspberry & Red Wine Crumble

Ingredients for 6 servings
2 cups raspberries
¼ cup red wine
1 teaspoon cinnamon
1 ¼ cup erythritol, divided
1 tsp vanilla extract
1 cup salted butter, cubed
1 ½ cups almond flour
¾ cup coconut flour

Directions and Total Time: approx. 55 minutes
Preheat oven 375 F. In a baking dish, add raspberries, red wine, half of erythritol, vanilla extract, and stir. In a bowl, rub butter with almond and coconut flours, and erythritol until it resembles large breadcrumbs. Spoon the mixture to cover the raspberries, place in the oven, and bake for 45 minutes until the top is golden brown. Cool and serve.
Per serving: Cal 318; Net Carbs 4.8g, Fat 31g, Protein 1.5g

Avocado Fries

Ingredients for 2 servings
½ cup olive oil
3 avocados, sliced
1 ½ tbsp almond flour
Salt and black pepper to taste
1 cup grated Parmesan cheese
2 large eggs, beaten in a bowl

Directions and Total Time: approx. 10 minutes
In a bowl, combine flour, salt, pepper, and Parmesan. Toss avocado slices in eggs and then dredge in the Parmesan mixture. Heat olive oil in a deep pan. Fry avocado slices until golden brown, 2 minutes, and transfer to a wire rack.
Per serving: Cal 849; Net Carbs 7.2g; Fat 77g; Protein 21g

Cacao Nut Bites

Ingredients for 4 servings
3 ½ oz dark chocolate
½ cup mixed nuts
2 tbsp roasted coconut chips
1 tbsp sunflower seeds
Directions and Total Time: approx. 5 minutes
Microwave chocolate for 2 minutes. Into 10 small cupcake liners, share the chocolate. Drop in nuts, coconut chips, sunflower seeds and sprinkle with salt. Chill until firm.
Per serving: Cal 72; Net Carbs 3g; Fat 5g; Protein 2g

Cranberry Coconut Parfait

Ingredients for 4 servings
2 cups coconut yogurt
¼ cup fresh cranberries
½ lemon, zested
3 mint sprigs, chopped
2 tbsp hemp seeds
Sugar-free maple syrup to taste
Directions and Total Time: approx. 5 minutes
In serving glasses, add half of coconut yogurt, cranberries, lemon zest, mint, hemp seeds, and drizzle with maple syrup. Repeat a second layer. Serve with maple syrup.
Per serving: Cal 105; Net Carbs 2.9g, Fat 7.8g, Protein 5g

SNACKS & SIDE DISHES

Jalapeño Nacho Wings

Ingredients for 4 servings
2 cups shredded Mexican cheese blend
16 chicken wings, halved
½ cup butter, melted
1 cup golden flaxseed meal
2 tbsp chopped green chilies
1 cup chopped scallions
1 jalapeño pepper, sliced

Directions and Total Time: approx. 45 minutes
Preheat oven to 350 F. Toss chicken with butter, salt, pepper to coat. Spread the flaxseed meal in a wide plate and roll in each chicken wing. Place on a baking sheet and bake for 30-35 minutes or until golden brown and cooked within. Sprinkle with the cheese blend, green chilies, scallions, and jalapeño pepper on top. Serve immediately.
Per serving: Cal 798; Net Carbs 1.5g; Fat 61g; Protein 48g

Easy Bacon & Cheese Balls

Ingredients for 4 servings
7 bacon slices, chopped
6 oz cream cheese
6 oz shredded Gruyere cheese
2 tbsp butter, softened
½ tsp red chili flakes

Directions and Total Time: approx. 30 minutes
Put bacon in a skillet and fry over medium heat until crispy, 5 minutes. Transfer to a plate, crumble after. Pour the bacon grease into a bowl and mix in cream cheese, Gruyere cheese, butter, and red chili flakes. Refrigerate to set for 15 minutes. Remove and mold into walnut-sized balls. Roll in the crumbled bacon. Plate and serve.
Per serving: Cal 538; Net Carbs 0.5g; Fat 50g; Protein 22g

Chili Turnip Fries

Ingredients for 4 servings
6 large parsnips, sliced
3 tbsp ground pork rinds
3 tbsp olive oil
¼ tsp red chili flakes

Directions and Total Time: approx. 50 minutes
Preheat oven to 425 F. Pour parsnips into a bowl and add in pork rinds, salt, and pepper. Toss and divide the parsnips between 2 baking sheets. Drizzle with olive oil and sprinkle with chili flakes. Bake in the oven until crispy, 40 to 45 minutes, tossing halfway. Serve.
Per serving: Cal 260; Net Carbs 22.6g; Fat 11g; Protein 3g

Baked Toast Strips with Prosciutto Butter

Ingredients for 4 servings

4 slices prosciutto, chopped
2 shallots
½ cup butter, softened
1 tbsp fresh basil
1 tsp tomato paste
4 slices zero carb bread
2 tbsp extra-virgin olive oil

Directions and Total Time: approx. 0 minutes

Add prosciutto, 1 tbsp of butter, and shallots to a skillet. Cook with frequent stirring for 5 minutes; let cool. Mix in the remaining butter, basil, and tomato paste. Season with salt and pepper. Spoon into a bowl and chill for 30 minutes to solidify slightly. Brush zero carb bread with olive oil, cut into strips, place on a baking sheet and toast for 3-5 minutes in a preheated at 400 F oven or until brown and crispy. Sprinkle with salt, and serve with prosciutto butter.
Per serving: Cal 315; Net Carbs 8.8g; Fat 28g; Protein 5g

Cauliflower Rice & Bacon Gratin

Ingredients for 4 servings

1 cup canned artichoke hearts, drained and chopped
6 bacon slices, chopped
2 cups cauliflower rice
3 cups baby spinach, chopped
1 garlic clove, minced
1 tbsp olive oil
Salt and black pepper to taste
¼ cup sour cream
8 oz cream cheese, softened
¼ cup grated Parmesan
1 ½ cups grated mozzarella

Directions and Total Time: approx. 30 minutes

Preheat oven to 350 F. Cook bacon in a skillet over medium heat until brown and crispy, 5 minutes. Spoon onto a plate. In a bowl, mix cauli rice, artichokes, spinach, garlic, olive oil, salt, pepper, sour cream, cream cheese, bacon, and half of Parmesan cheese. Spread the mixture into a baking dish and top with the remaining Parmesan and mozzarella cheeses. Bake 15 minutes. Serve.
Per serving: Cal 500; Net Carbs 5.3g; Fat 37g; Protein 28g

Crunchy Rutabaga Puffs

Ingredients for 4 servings
1 rutabaga, peeled and diced
2 tbsp melted butter
½ oz goat cheese
¼ cup ground pork rinds

Directions and Total Time: approx. 35 minutes
Preheat oven to 400 F and spread rutabaga on a baking sheet. Season with salt, pepper, and drizzle with the butter. Bake until tender, 15 minutes. Transfer to a bowl. Allow cooling and add in goat cheese. Using a fork, mash and mix the ingredients. Pour the pork rinds onto a plate. Mold 1-inch balls out of the rutabaga mixture and roll properly in the rinds while pressing gently to stick. Place in the same baking sheet and bake for 10 minutes until golden.
Per serving: Cal 129; Net Carbs 5.9g; Fat 8g; Protein 3g

Crispy Pancetta & Butternut Squash Roast

Ingredients for 4 servings
2 butternut squash, cubed
1 tsp turmeric powder
½ tsp garlic powder
8 pancetta slices, chopped
2 tbsp olive oil
1 tbsp chopped cilantro,

Directions and Total Time: approx. 30 minutes
Preheat oven to 425 F. In a bowl, add butternut squash, salt, pepper, turmeric, garlic powder, pancetta, and olive oil. Toss until well-coated. Spread the mixture onto a greased baking sheet and roast for 10-15 minutes. Transfer the veggies to a bowl and garnish with cilantro to serve.
Per serving: Cal 148; Net Carbs 6.4g; Fat 10g; Protein 6g

Simple Stuffed Eggs with Mayonnaise

Ingredients for 6 servings
6 eggs
1 tbsp green tabasco
¼ cup mayonnaise
2 tbsp black olives, sliced

Directions and Total Time: approx. 30 minutes
Place eggs in a saucepan and cover with salted water. Boil for 10 minutes. Place the eggs in an ice bath and let cool. Peel and slice in half lengthwise. Scoop out the yolks to a bowl; mash with a fork. Whisk together the tabasco, mayonnaise, mashed yolks, and salt, in a bowl. Spoon this mixture into egg white. Garnish with olive slices to serve.
Per serving: Cal 178; Net Carbs: 5g; Fat: 17g; Protein: 6g

Cheesy Pork Rind Bread

Ingredients for 4 servings
¼ cup grated Pecorino Romano cheese
8 oz cream cheese
2 cups grated mozzarella
1 tbsp baking powder
1 cup crushed pork rinds
3 large eggs
1 tbsp Italian mixed herbs

Directions and Total Time: approx. 30 minutes
Preheat oven to 375 F and line a baking sheet with parchment paper. Microwave cream and mozzarella cheeses for 1 minute or until melted. Whisk in baking powder, pork rinds, eggs, Pecorino cheese, and mixed herbs. Spread the mixture in the baking sheet and bake for 20 minutes until lightly brown. Let cool, slice and serve.
Per serving: Cal 437; Net Carbs 3.2g; Fat 23g; Protein 32g

Savory Lime Fried Artichokes

Ingredients for 4 servings
12 fresh baby artichokes
2 tbsp lime juice
2 tbsp olive oil
Salt to taste

Directions and Total Time: approx. 20 minutes
Slice artichokes vertically into narrow wedges. Drain on paper towels before frying. Heat olive oil in a skillet. Fry the artichokes until browned and crispy. Drain excess oil on paper towels. Sprinkle with salt and lime juice.
Per serving: Cal 35; Net Carbs: 2.9g; Fat: 2.4g; Protein: 2g

Rosemary Cheese Chips with Guacamole

Ingredients for 4 servings
1 tbsp rosemary
1 cup Grana Padano, grated
¼ tsp sweet paprika
¼ tsp garlic powder
2 avocados, pitted and scooped
1 tomato, chopped

Directions and Total Time: approx. 20 minutes
Preheat oven to 350 F and line a baking sheet with parchment paper. Mix Grana Padano cheese, paprika, rosemary, and garlic powder evenly. Spoon 6-8 teaspoons on the baking sheet creating spaces between each mound.; flatten mounds. Bake for 5 minutes, cool, and remove to a plate. To make the guacamole, mash avocado, with a fork in a bowl, add in tomato and continue to mash until mostly smooth. Season with salt. Serve crackers with guacamole.
Per serving: Cal 229; Net Carbs 2g; Fat 20g; Protein 10g

Parmesan Green Bean Crisps

Ingredients for 6 servings
¼ cup Parmesan, shredded
¼ cup pork rind crumbs
1 tsp minced garlic
2 eggs
1 lb green beans
Salt and black pepper to taste

Directions and Total Time: approx. 30 minutes
Preheat oven to 425 F and line two baking sheets with foil. Mix Parmesan cheese, pork rinds, garlic, salt, and pepper in a bowl. Beat the eggs in another bowl. Coat green beans in eggs, then cheese mixture and arrange evenly on the baking sheets. Grease lightly with cooking spray and bake for 15 minutes. Transfer to a wire rack to cool. Serve.
Per serving: Cal 210; Net Carbs 3g; Fat 19g; Protein 5g

Paprika & Dill Deviled Eggs

Ingredients for 4 servings
1 tsp dill, chopped
8 large eggs
3 cups water
3 tbsp sriracha sauce
4 tbsp mayonnaise
¼ tsp sweet paprika

Directions and Total Time: approx. 20 minutes
Bring eggs to boil in salted water, reduce the heat, and simmer for 10 minutes. Transfer to an ice water bath, let cool completely and peel the shells. Slice the eggs in half height wise and empty the yolks into a bowl. Smash with a fork and mix in sriracha sauce, mayonnaise, and half of the paprika until smooth. Spoon filling into a piping bag and fill the egg whites to be slightly above the brim. Garnish with remaining paprika and dill and serve immediately.
Per serving: Cal 195; Net Carbs 1g; Fat 19g; Protein 4g

Cheese & Garlic Crackers

Ingredients for 6 servings
1 ¼ cups Pecorino Romano cheese, grated
1 ¼ cups coconut flour
Salt and black pepper to taste
1 tsp garlic powder
¼ cup ghee
¼ tsp sweet paprika
½ cup heavy cream

Directions and Total Time: approx. 30 minutes
Preheat oven to 350 F. Mix flour, Pecorino Romano cheese, salt, pepper, garlic and paprika in a bowl. Add in ghee and mix well. Top with heavy cream and mix again until a thick mixture has formed. Cover the dough with plastic wrap. Use a rolling pin to spread out the dough into a light rectangle. Cut into cracker squares and arrange them on a baking sheet. Bake for 20 minutes.
Per serving: Cal 115; Net Carbs 0.7g; Fat 3g; Protein 5g

Cheesy Chicken Wraps

Ingredients for 8 servings
¼ tsp garlic powder
8 ounces fontina cheese
8 raw chicken tenders
8 prosciutto slices

Directions and Total Time: approx. 20 minutes
Pound chicken until half an inch thick. Season with garlic powder. Cut fontina cheese into 8 strips. Place a slice of prosciutto on a flat surface. Place one chicken tender on top. Top with a fontina strip. Roll the chicken and secure with skewers. Grill the wraps for 3 minutes per side.
Per serving: Cal 174; Net Carbs: 0.7g; Fat: 10g; Protein: 17g

Baked Chorizo with Cottage Cheese

Ingredients for 6 servings
7 oz Spanish chorizo, sliced
4 oz cottage cheese, pureed
¼ cup chopped parsley

Directions and Total Time: approx. 30 minutes
Preheat the oven to 325 F. Line a baking dish with waxed paper. Bake the chorizo for 15 minutes until crispy. Remove from the oven and let cool. Arrange on a serving platter. Top each slice with cottage cheese and parsley.
Per serving: Cal 172; Net Carbs: 0.2g; Fat: 13g; Protein: 5g

Goat Cheese Stuffed Peppers

Ingredients for 8 servings
8 canned roasted piquillo peppers
3 slices prosciutto, cut into thin slices
2 tbsp olive oil
8 ounces goat cheese
3 tbsp heavy cream
3 tbsp chopped parsley
½ tsp minced garlic
1 tbsp chopped mint

Directions and Total Time: approx. 15 minutes
Combine goat cheese, heavy cream, parsley, garlic, and mint in a bowl. Place the mixture in a freezer bag, press down and squeeze, and cut off the bottom. Drain and deseed the peppers. Squeeze about 2 tbsp of the filling into each pepper. Wrap a prosciutto slice onto each pepper. Secure with toothpicks. Arrange them on a serving platter. Sprinkle the olive oil and vinegar over.
Per serving: Cal 110; Net Carbs 2.5g; Fat 9g; Protein 6g

Fried Artichoke Hearts

Ingredients for 4 servings
12 fresh baby artichokes
2 tbsp lemon juice
3 tbsp olive oil
Salt to taste

Directions and Total Time: approx. 15 minutes
Slice the artichokes vertically into narrow wedges. Drain them on a piece of paper towel before frying. Heat olive oil in a cast-iron skillet over high heat. Fry the artichokes until browned and crispy. Drain excess oil, sprinkle with salt and lemon juice.
Per serving: Cal 35; Net Carbs 2.9g; Fat 2.4g; Protein 2g

Provolone & Prosciutto Chicken Wraps

Ingredients for 8 servings
¼ tsp garlic powder
8 ounces provolone cheese
8 chicken tenders
8 prosciutto slices

Directions and Total Time: approx. 20 minutes
Pound the chicken until half an inch thick. Season with garlic powder. Cut the provolone cheese into 8 strips. Place a slice of prosciutto on a flat surface. Place one chicken tender on top. Top with a provolone strip. Roll the chicken and secure with previously soaked skewers. Grill the wraps for about 3 minutes per side.
Per serving: Cal 174; Net Carbs 0.7g; Fat 10g; Protein 17g

Tuna Topped Pickles

Ingredients for 8 servings
12 oz smoked canned tuna
6 large dill pickles, halved
¼ tsp garlic powder
⅓ cup sugar-free mayonnaise
1 tbsp onion flakes

Directions and Total Time: approx. 40 minutes
Combine the seasonings, mayonnaise, and tuna in a bowl. Top each pickle half with the tuna mixture. Place in the fridge for 30 minutes before serving.
Per serving: Cal 118; Net Carbs 1.5g; Fat 10g; Protein 11g

Keto Deviled Eggs

Ingredients for 6 servings
6 eggs
1 tbsp green tabasco
⅓ cup sugar-free mayonnaise Salt to taste

Directions and Total Time: approx. 30 minutes
Place eggs in a saucepan and cover with salted water. Bring to a boil over medium heat, for 8 minutes. Place in an ice bath to cool. Peel and slice. Whisk tabasco, mayo, and salt, in a bowl. Top every egg with some mayo dressing.
Per serving: Cal 178; Net Carbs 5g; Fat 17g; Protein 6g

Bacon & Pistachio Liverwurst Truffles

Ingredients for 8 servings
8 bacon slices, cooked and chopped
8 ounces liverwurst
¼ cup chopped pistachios
1 tsp Dijon mustard
6 ounces cream cheese

Directions and Total Time: approx. 45 minutes
Combine liverwurst and pistachios in a food processor. Pulse until smooth. Whisk cream cheese and mustard in another bowl. Make 12 balls out of the liverwurst mixture. Make a thin cream cheese layer over. Coat with bacon pieces. Arrange on a plate and refrigerate for 30 minutes.
Per serving: Cal 145; Net Carbs 1.5g; Fat 12g; Protein 7g

Baked Spicy Eggplants

Ingredients for 4 servings
2 large eggplants
2 tbsp butter
1 tsp red chili flakes
4 oz raw ground almonds

Directions and Total Time: approx. 30 minutes
Preheat oven to 400 F. Cut off the head of the eggplants and slice the body into rounds. Arrange on a parchment paper-lined baking sheet. Drop thin slices of butter on each eggplant slice, sprinkle with chili flakes, and bake for 20 minutes. Slide out and sprinkle with almonds. Roast further for 5 minutes. Serve with arugula salad.
Per serving: Cal 230; Net Carbs 4g; Fat 16g; Protein 14g

Mashed Broccoli with Roasted Garlic

Ingredients for 4 servings
1 large head broccoli, cut into florets
½ head garlic
2 tbsp olive oil
4 oz butter
¼ tsp dried thyme
Juice and zest of half a lemon
4 tbsp coconut cream
4 tbsp olive oil

Directions and Total Time: approx. 45 minutes
Preheat oven to 400 F. Wrap garlic in aluminum foil and roast for 30 minutes; set aside. Pour broccoli into a pot and cover with salted water. Bring to a boil over high heat until tender, about 7 minutes. Drain and transfer to a bowl. Add in butter, thyme, lemon juice and zest, coconut cream, and olive oil. Use an immersion blender to puree the ingredients until smooth. Serve drizzled with olive oil.
Per serving: Cal 376; Net Carbs 6g; Fat 33g; Protein 11g

Spicy Pistachio Dip

Ingredients for 4 servings
3 oz toasted pistachios
3 tbsp coconut cream
¼ cup water
Juice of half a lemon
½ tsp smoked paprika
Cayenne pepper to taste
½ tsp salt
½ cup olive oil

Directions and Total Time: approx. 5 minutes
Pour pistachios, cream, water, lemon juice, paprika, cayenne, and salt in a food processor. Puree until smooth. Add in olive oil and puree again. Spoon into bowls, garnish with pistachios, and serve with celery and carrots.
Per serving: Cal 220; Net Carbs 5g; Fat 19g; Protein 6g

Prosciutto Appetizer with Blackberries

Ingredients for 4 servings
4 zero carb bread slices
¾ cup balsamic vinegar
2 tbsp erythritol
1 cup fresh blackberries
1 cup crumbled goat cheese
¼ tsp dry Italian seasoning
1 tbsp almond milk
4 thin prosciutto slices

Directions and Total Time: approx. 25 minutes
Cut the bread into 3 pieces each and arrange on a baking sheet. Place under the broiler and toast for 1-2 minutes on each side or until golden brown; set aside. In a saucepan, add balsamic vinegar and stir in erythritol until dissolved. Boil the mixture over medium heat until reduced by half, 5 minutes. Turn the heat off and carefully stir in the blackberries. Make sure they do not break open. Set aside.In a bowl, add goat cheese, Italian seasoning, and almond milk. Mix until smooth. Brush one side of the toasted bread with the balsamic reduction and top with the cheese mixture. Cut each prosciutto slice into 3 pieces and place on the bread. Top with some of the whole blackberries from the balsamic mixture. Serve immediately.
Per serving: Cal 175; Net Carbs 8.7g; Fat 7g; Protein 18g

Onion Rings & Kale Dip

Ingredients for 4 servings
1 onion, sliced in rings
1 tbsp flax seed meal
1 cup almond flour
½ cup grated Parmesan
1 tsp garlic powder
½ tbsp sweet paprika powder
2 oz chopped kale
2 tbsp olive oil
2 tbsp dried cilantro
1 tbsp dried oregano
Salt and black pepper to taste
1 cup mayonnaise
4 tbsp coconut cream
Juice of ½ lemon

Directions and Total Time: approx. 35 minutes
Preheat oven to 400 F. In a bowl, mix flax seed meal and 3 tbsp water and leave the mixture to thicken and fully absorb for 5 minutes. In another bowl, combine almond flour, Parmesan cheese, garlic powder, paprika, and salt. Line a baking sheet with parchment paper. When the flax egg is ready, dip in the onion rings one after another, and then into the almond flour mixture. Place the rings on the sheet and spray with cooking spray. Bake for 20 minutes. Remove to a bowl. Put kale in a bowl. Add in olive oil, cilantro, oregano, salt, pepper, mayonnaise, coconut cream, and lemon juice; mix well. Let sit for 10 minutes. Serve the dip with the crispy onion rings.
Per serving: Cal 410; Net Carbs 7g; Fat 35g; Protein 14g

Paprika Roasted Nuts

Ingredients for 4 servings
8 oz walnuts and pecans
1 tbsp coconut oil
1 tsp cumin powder
1 tsp paprika powder

Directions and Total Time: approx. 10 minutes
In a bowl, mix walnuts, pecans, salt, coconut oil, cumin powder, and paprika powder until the nuts are well coated. Pour the mixture into a frying pan and toast over medium heat while stirring continually until fragrant and brown.
Per serving: Cal 290; Net Carbs 3g; Fat 27g; Protein 6g

Mediterranean Deviled Eggs

Ingredients for 6 servings
6 large eggs
Ice water bath
1 tsp Dijon mustard
3 tbsp mayonnaise
1 tsp white wine vinegar
2 tbsp crumbled feta cheese
¼ tsp turmeric powder
1 red chili, minced
1 tbsp chopped parsley
Smoked paprika to garnish

Directions and Total Time: approx. 30 minutes
Boil eggs in salted water for 10 minutes. Transfer to an ice water bath. Let cool for 5 minutes, peel and slice in half. Remove the yolks to a bowl and put the whites on a plate. Mash yolks with a fork and mix in mustard, mayonnaise, vinegar, feta, turmeric, and chili until evenly combined. Spoon the mixture into a piping bag and fill into the egg whites. Garnish with parsley and paprika. Serve.
Per serving: Cal 139; Net Carbs 1.2g, Fat 8.2g, Protein 7g

Mushroom Broccoli Faux Risotto

Ingredients for 4 servings
1 cup cremini mushrooms, chopped
4 oz butter
2 garlic cloves, minced
1 red onion, finely chopped
1 head broccoli, grated
1 cup water
¾ cup white wine
Salt and black pepper to taste
1 cup coconut cream
¾ cup grated Parmesan
Freshly chopped thyme

Directions and Total Time: approx. 25 minutes
Place a pot over medium heat and melt butter. Sauté mushrooms until golden, 5 minutes. Add in garlic and onions and cook for 3 minutes until fragrant and soft. Mix in broccoli, water, and half of white wine. Season with salt and pepper and simmer for 10 minutes. Mix in coconut cream and simmer until most of the cream evaporates. Turn heat off and stir in Parmesan and thyme. Serve warm.
Per serving: Cal 520; Net Carbs 12g; Fat 43g; Protein 15g

Spinach Chips with Guacamole Hummus

Ingredients for 4 servings
½ cup baby spinach
1 tbsp olive oil
½ tsp plain vinegar
3 avocados, chopped
½ cup chopped parsley
½ cup butter
¼ cup pumpkin seeds
¼ cup sesame paste
Juice from ½ lemon
1 garlic clove, minced
½ tsp coriander powder
Salt and black pepper to taste

Directions and Total Time: approx. 30 minutes
Preheat oven to 300 F. Put spinach in a bowl and toss with olive oil, plain vinegar, and salt. Arrange on a parchment paper-lined baking sheet and bake until the leaves are crispy but not burned, 15 minutes. Place avocado to a food processor. Add in butter, pumpkin seeds, sesame paste, lemon juice, garlic, coriander, salt, and pepper; puree until smooth. Spoon into a bowl and garnish with parsley. Serve with the spinach chips.
Per serving: Cal 473; Net Carbs 3g; Fat 45g; Protein 8g

Tofu Stuffed Peppers

Ingredients for 4 servings
2 red bell peppers
1 cup grated Parmesan
1 oz tofu, chopped
1 tbsp fresh parsley, chopped
1 cup cream cheese
1 tbsp chili paste, mild
2 tbsp melted butter

Directions and Total Time: approx. 25 minutes
Preheat oven to 400 F. Cut bell peppers into two, lengthwise and remove the core and seeds. In a bowl, mix tofu with parsley, cream cheese, chili paste, and melted butter until smooth. Spoon the cheese mixture into the bell peppers. Arrange peppers on a greased sheet. Sprinkle Parmesan on top and bake for 20 minutes.
Per serving: Cal 412; Net Carbs 5g; Fat 36g; Protein 14g

Soy Chorizo Stuffed Cabbage Rolls

Ingredients for 4 servings
¼ cup coconut oil
1 onion, chopped
3 cloves garlic, minced
1 cup crumbled soy chorizo
1 cup cauliflower rice
1 can tomato sauce
1 tsp dried oregano
1 tsp dried basil
Salt and black pepper to taste
8 full green cabbage leaves

Directions and Total Time: approx. 35 minutes
Heat coconut oil in a saucepan and add onion, garlic, and soy chorizo; sauté for 5 minutes. Stir in cauli rice, season with salt and pepper, and cook for 4 minutes; set aside. In the saucepan, pour tomato sauce, season with salt, pepper, oregano, and basil. Add ¼ cup of water and simmer the sauce for 10 minutes. Lay cabbage leaves on a flat surface and spoon the soy chorizo mixture into the middle of each leaf. Roll the leaves to secure the filling. Place the cabbage rolls in the tomato sauce and cook for 10 minutes.
Per serving: Cal 285; Net Carbs 7g; Fat 26g; Protein 5g

Cauliflower Chips with Cheese Dip

Ingredients for 6 servings
1 head cauliflower, cut into florets
¾ cup dried cranberries, chopped
½ cup toasted pecans, chopped
1 ½ tbsp almond flour
1 tbsp flax seeds
4 tbsp chia seeds
8 oz cream cheese, softened
2 tbsp sugar-free maple syrup
1 tbsp lemon zest

Directions and Total Time: approx. 35 minutes
Preheat oven to 350 F. Pour cauliflower and 2 cups salted water in a pot and bring to a boil for 5 minutes. Drain and transfer to a food processor; puree until very smooth. Pour into a bowl and stir in flour until evenly combined. Mix in flax seeds and 1 tbsp chia seeds. Line a large baking sheet with parchment paper and spread in the batter. Cover with a plastic wrap and use a rolling pin to flatten and level the mixture evenly and lightly. Take off the plastic wrap and use cut our chip-size squares on the batter. Bake for 20 minutes or until the chips are golden brown and crispy. Let cool for 5 minutes and transfer to a serving bowl. In a bowl, mix cream cheese with maple syrup until properly mixed. Add in cranberries, pecans, remaining chia seeds, and lemon juice; mix well. Serve the dip with cauli chips.

Mozzarella in Prosciutto Blanket

Ingredients for 6 servings
18 mozzarella cheese ciliegine
6 thin prosciutto slices
18 basil leaves

Directions and Total Time: approx. 15 minutes
Cut the prosciutto slices into three strips. Place basil leaves at the end of each strip. Top with mozzarella. Wrap the mozzarella in prosciutto. Secure with toothpicks. Serve.
Per serving: Cal 163; Net Carbs 0.2g; Fat 12g; Protein 13g
Per serving: Cal 252; Net Carbs 6.2g; Fat 23g; Protein 6g

Chocolate, Berries & Nut Mix Bars

Ingredients for 4 servings
¼ cup walnuts
¼ cup cashew nuts
¼ cup almonds
¼ cup coconut chips
1 egg, beaten
½ cup butter, melted
¼ cup dark chocolate chips
¼ cup mixed seeds
Salt to taste
1 cup mixed dried berries

Directions and Total Time: approx. 25 minutes
Preheat oven to 350 F and line a baking sheet with parchment paper. In a food processor, pulse nuts until roughly chopped. Place in a bowl; stir in chips, egg, butter, mixed seeds, salt, and berries. Spread the mixture in the sheet and bake for 18 minutes. Let cool and cut into bars.
Per serving: Cal 384; Net Carbs 6.4g; Fat 37.7g; Protein 6g

Chili Avocado-Chimichurri Appetizer

Ingredients for 4 servings
4 zero carb bread slices
¼ cup + 2 tbsp olive oil
2 tbsp red wine vinegar
1 lemon, juiced
Salt and black pepper to taste
3 garlic cloves, minced
½ tsp red chili flakes
½ tsp dried oregano
½ cup chopped fresh parsley
2 avocados, cubed

Directions and Total Time: approx. 15 minutes
Cut bread slices in half, brush both sides with 2 tbsp of the olive oil, and arrange on a baking sheet. Place under the broiler and toast for 1-2 minutes per side. In a bowl, mix the remaining olive oil, vinegar, lemon juice, salt, pepper, garlic, red chili flakes, oregano, and parsley. Fold in the avocados Spoon the mixture onto the bread and serve.
Per serving: Cal 305; Net Carbs 5.6g; Fat 26g; Protein 9g

Crispy Squash Nacho Chips

Ingredients for 4 servings
1 yellow squash, sliced
Salt to season
1 ½ cups coconut oil
1 tbsp taco seasoning

Directions and Total Time: approx. 25 minutes
Pour coconut oil in a skillet and heat oil over medium heat. Add in squash slices and fry until crispy and golden brown. Remove to a paper towel-lined plate. Sprinkle the slices with taco seasoning and salt and serve.
Per serving: Cal 150; Net Carbs 1g; Fat 14g; Protein 2g

Chocolate Walnut Biscuits

Ingredients for 4 servings
2/3 cup dark chocolate chips
4 oz butter, softened
2 tbsp swerve sugar
2 tbsp swerve brown sugar
1 egg
1 tsp vanilla extract
½ cup almond flour
½ tsp baking soda
½ cup chopped walnuts

Directions and Total Time: approx. 30 minutes
Preheat oven to 350 F. In a bowl, whisk butter, swerve sugar, and swerve until smooth. Beat in the egg and mix in the vanilla extract. In another bowl, combine almond flour with baking soda and mix into the wet ingredients. Fold in chocolate chips and walnuts. Spoon tablespoons full of the batter onto a greased baking sheet, creating 2-inch spaces in between each spoon, and press down each dough to slightly flatten. Bake for 15 minutes. Transfer to a wire rack to cool completely. Serve.
Per serving: Cal 430; Net Carbs 3.5g; Fat 42g; Protein 6g

Herby Cheesy Nuts

Ingredients for 4 servings
1 egg white
4 tsp yeast extract
1 tsp swerve brown sugar
1 ½ cups mixed nuts
½ cup mixed seeds
Salt and black pepper to taste
3 tbsp grated Parmesan
½ tsp dried mixed herbs

Directions and Total Time: approx. 20 minutes
Preheat oven to 350 F. In a bowl, beat egg white, yeast extract, and swerve. Add in mixed nuts and seeds; combine and spread onto a baking sheet. Bake for 10 minutes. In a bowl, mix salt, pepper, Parmesan, and herbs. Remove the nuts and toss with the cheese mixture. Bake for 5 minutes until sticky and brown. Let cool for 5 minutes and serve.
Per serving: Cal 494; Net Carbs 6g; Fat 48g; Protein 11g

Mixed Seed Crackers

Ingredients for 6 servings
1/3 cup sesame seed flour
1/3 cup pumpkin seeds
1/3 cup sunflower seeds
1/3 cup sesame seeds
1/3 cup chia seeds
1 tbsp psyllium husk powder
1 tsp salt
¼ cup butter, melted

Directions and Total Time: approx. 60 minutes
Preheat oven to 300 F. Combine sesame seed flour with pumpkin, chia and sunflower seeds, psyllium husk powder, and salt. Pour in butter and 1 cup boiling water and mix until a dough forms with a gel-like consistency. Line a baking sheet with parchment paper and place the dough on the sheet. Cover with another parchment paper and with a rolling pin to flatten into the baking sheet. Remove the parchment paper on top. Bake for 45 minutes. Turn off and allow the crackers to cool and dry in the oven, 10 minutes. Break and serve.
Per serving: Cal 65; Net Carbs 2g; Fat 5g; Protein 3g

Cheddar and Halloumi Sticks

Ingredients for 6 servings
1/3 cup almond flour
2 tsp smoked paprika
1 lb halloumi, cut into strips
½ cup grated cheddar cheese
2 tbsp chopped parsley
½ tsp cayenne powder

Directions and Total Time: approx. 15 minutes
Preheat oven to 350 F. In a bowl, mix flour with paprika and lightly dredge the halloumi cheese in the mixture. Arrange on a greased baking sheet. In a smaller bowl, combine parsley, cheddar cheese, and cayenne. Sprinkle the mixture on the cheese and lightly grease with cooking spray. Bake for 10 minutes until golden brown. Serve.
Per serving: Cal 886; Net Carbs 6.1g; Fat 77g; Protein 14g

Pesto Mushroom Pinwheels

Ingredients for 4 servings
¼ cup almond flour
3 tbsp coconut flour
½ tsp xanthan gum
4 tbsp cream cheese, softened
1/4 teaspoon yogurt
¼ cup butter, cold
3 whole eggs
3 tbsp erythritol
1 ½ tsp vanilla extract
1 whole egg, beaten
1 cup mushrooms, chopped
1 cup basil pesto
2 cups baby spinach
Salt and black pepper to taste
1 cup grated cheddar cheese
1 egg, beaten for brushing

Directions and Total Time: approx. 40 minutes
In a bowl, mix almond and coconut flours, xanthan gum, and ½ tsp salt. Add in yogurt, cream cheese, and butter; mix until crumbly. Add in erythritol and vanilla extract until mixed. Pour in 3 eggs one after another while mixing until formed into a ball. Flatten the dough on a clean flat surface, cover in plastic wrap, and refrigerate for 1 hour. Dust a clean flat surface with almond flour, unwrap the dough, and roll out into 15x12 inches. Spread pesto on top with a spatula, leaving a 2-inch border on one end. In a bowl, combine baby spinach and mushrooms, season with salt and pepper, and spread the mixture over pesto. Sprinkle with cheddar cheese and roll up as tightly as possible from the shorter end. Refrigerate for 10 minutes. Preheat oven to 380 F. Remove the pastry onto a flat surface and use a sharp knife to into 24 slim discs. Arrange on the baking sheet, brush with the remaining egg, and bake for 25 minutes until golden. Let cool for 5 minutes.
Per serving: Cal 535; Net Carbs 4g; Fat 41g; Protein 34.6g

Hemp Seed Zucchini Chips

Ingredients for 4 servings
4 large zucchinis, sliced
4 tbsp olive oil
1 tsp smoked paprika
2 tbsp hemp seeds
2 tbsp poppy seeds
1 tsp red chili flakes

Directions and Total Time: approx. 15 minutes
Preheat oven to 350 F. Drizzle zucchini with olive oil and sprinkle with paprika. Scatter with the hemp seeds, poppy seeds, and chili flakes. Season with salt, pepper, and roast for 20 minutes or until crispy and golden brown. Serve.
Per serving: Cal 173; Net Carbs 1.3g; Fat 18g; Protein 2.2g

All Seeds Flapjacks

Ingredients for 4 servings
4 tbsp dried goji berries, chopped
6 tbsp salted butter
8 tbsp sugar-free maple syrup
8 tbsp swerve brown sugar
3 tbsp sesame seeds
3 tbsp chia seeds
3 tbsp hemp seeds
3 tbsp sunflower seeds
1 tbsp poppy seeds

Directions and Total Time: approx. 30 minutes
Preheat oven to 350 F and line a baking sheet with parchment paper. Place butter, maple syrup, and swerve brown sugar in a saucepan over low heat, stir in swerve brown sugar until dissolved. Remove and stir all seeds along with goji berries until evenly combined. Spread into the baking sheet and bake for 20 minutes or until golden brown. Slice flapjacks into the 16 strips. Serve.
Per serving: Cal 300; Net Carbs 3g; Fat 28g; Protein 6.8g

Tasty Keto Snickerdoodles

Ingredients for 4 servings
2 cups almond flour
½ tsp baking soda
¾ cup sweetener
½ cup butter, softened
2 tbsp erythritol sweetener
1 tsp cinnamon

Directions and Total Time: approx. 25 minutes
Preheat oven to 350 F. Combine almond flour, baking soda, sweetener, and butter in a bowl. Make 16 balls out of the mixture. Flatten them with your hands. Combine the cinnamon and erythritol in a bowl. Dip in the cookies and arrange on a lined cookie sheet. Bake for 15 minutes.
Per serving: Cal 131; Net Carbs 1.5g; Fat 13g; Protein 3g

Basil-Chili Mozzarella Bites

Ingredients for 4 servings
1 cup olive oil, for frying
1 cup almond flour
½ tsp chili powder
1 tsp onion powder
1 tsp garlic powder
1 tsp dried basil leaves
1 large egg, beaten in a bowl
1 cup golden flaxseed meal
1 cup mozzarella cheese cubes
¼ cup small tomatoes, halved
A handful of basil leaves

Directions and Total Time: approx. 10 minutes
In a bowl, combine flour, chili, onion and garlic powders, and basil; set aside. Pour flaxseed meal in a plate. Coat each cheese cube in the flour mixture, then in the egg, and then lightly in the golden flaxseed meal. Heat olive oil in a deep pan. Fry the cheese until golden brown on both sides. Transfer to a wire rack to drain grease. On each tomato half, place 1 basil leaf, top with a cheese cube, and insert a toothpick at the middle of the sandwich to hold. Serve.
Per serving: Cal 769; Net Carbs 2.4g; Fat 73g; Protein 18g

DESSERTS

Heart-Shaped Red Velvet Cakes

Ingredients for 6 servings
½ cup butter
6 eggs
1 tsp vanilla extract
1 cup Greek yogurt
1 cup swerve sugar
1 cup almond flour
½ cup coconut flour
2 tbsp cocoa powder
2 tbsp baking powder
¼ tsp salt
1 tbsp red food coloring

For the frosting:
1 cup mascarpone cheese
½ cup erythritol
1 tsp vanilla extract
2 tbsp heavy cream

Directions and Total Time: approx. 30 minutes
Preheat oven to 400 F and grease 2 heart-shaped cake pans with butter. In a bowl, beat butter, eggs, vanilla, Greek yogurt, and swerve sugar until smooth. In another bowl, mix the almond and coconut flours, cocoa, salt, baking powder, and red food coloring. Combine both mixtures until smooth and divide the batter between the two cake pans. Bake in the oven for 25 minutes or until a toothpick inserted comes out clean. Meanwhile, in a bowl, using an electric mixer, whisk the mascarpone cheese and erythritol until smooth. Mix in vanilla and heavy cream until well-combined. Transfer to a wire rack, let cool, and spread the frosting on top. Slice and serve.
Per serving: Cal 643; Net Carbs 9.2g; Fat 46g; Protein 37g

Chocolate Crunch Bars

Ingredients for 4 servings
1 ½ cups chocolate chips
¼ cup almond butter
½ cup sugar-free maple syrup
¼ cup melted butter
2 cups mixed seeds
1 cup chopped walnuts

Directions and Total Time: approx. 5 min + chilling time
Line a baking sheet with parchment paper. In a bowl, mix chips, almond butter, maple syrup, butter, seeds, and walnuts. Spread the mixture onto the sheet and refrigerate until firm, at least 1 hour. Cut into bars and enjoy.
Per serving: Cal 713; Net Carbs 7.1g; Fat 75g; Protein 7.9g

Sticky Maple Cinnamon Cake

Ingredients for 4 servings
9 tbsp butter, melted and cooled
½ cup sugar-free maple syrup + extra for topping
6 eggs
2 tsp cream cheese, softened
1 tsp vanilla extract
2 tbsp heavy cream
¼ cup almond flour
1 ½ tsp baking powder
1 tsp cinnamon powder
½ tsp salt

Directions and Total Time: approx. 30 minutes
Preheat oven to 400 F; grease a cake pan with melted butter. In a bowl, beat the eggs, butter, cream cheese, vanilla, heavy cream, and maple syrup until smooth. In another bowl, mix almond flour, baking powder, cinnamon, and salt. Combine both mixtures until smooth and pour the batter into the cake pan. Bake for 25 minutes or until a toothpick inserted comes out clean. Transfer the cake to a wire rack to cool and drizzle with maple syrup.
Per serving: Cal 362; Net Carbs 1.5g; Fat 35g; Protein 8.9g

Almond Square Cookies

Ingredients for 4 servings
2 ¼ cups almond flour
1 tsp baking powder
½ tsp salt
1 cup butter, softened
1 cup swerve sugar
1 large egg
¾ tsp almond extract

Directions and Total Time: approx. 30 minutes
Preheat oven to 400 F; line a baking sheet with parchment paper. In a bowl, mix almond flour, baking powder, and salt. In another bowl, mix butter, swerve, egg, and almond extract until well smooth. Combine both mixtures until smooth dough forms. Lay a parchment paper on a flat surface, place the dough and cover with another parchment paper. Using a rolling pin, flatten it into ½-inch thickness and cut it into squares. Arrange on the baking sheet with 1-inch intervals and bake in the oven until the edges are set and golden brown, 25 minutes.
Per serving: Cal 426; Net Carbs 0.4g; Fat 46g; Protein 1.4g

White Chocolate Chip Cookies

Ingredients for 4 servings
3 oz unsweetened white chocolate chips
½ cup unsalted butter
¾ cup xylitol
1 tsp vanilla extract
1 large egg
1 ½ cups almond flour
½ tsp baking powder
½ tsp xanthan gum
¼ tsp salt

Directions and Total Time: approx. 25 minutes
Preheat oven to 350 F; line a baking sheet with parchment paper. In a bowl and using an electric mixer, cream the butter and xylitol until light and fluffy. Add vanilla, egg, and beat until smooth. Add almond flour, baking powder, xanthan gum, salt, and whisk the mixture until smooth dough forms. Fold in chocolate chips. Roll the dough into 1 ½-inch balls and arrange on the sheet at 2-inch intervals. Bake for 12 minutes until lightly golden.
Per serving: Cal 163; Net Carbs 0.3g; Fat 16g; Protein 2.6g

Cowboy Cookies

Ingredients for 8 servings
1 cup butter, softened
1 cup swerve white sugar
1 cup swerve brown sugar
1 tbsp vanilla extract
2 large eggs
2 cups almond flour
2 tsp baking powder
1 tsp baking soda
1 tbsp cinnamon powder
1 tsp salt
1 cup sugar-free chocolate chips
1 cup peanut butter chips
2 cups golden flaxseed meal
1 ½ cups coconut flakes
2 cups chopped walnuts

Directions and Total Time: approx. 30 minutes
Preheat oven to 375 F; line a baking sheet with parchment paper. In a large bowl and using a hand mixer, cream the butter and swerve until light and fluffy. Slowly, beat in the vanilla and eggs until smooth. In a separate bowl, mix almond flour, baking powder, baking soda, cinnamon, and salt. Combine both mixtures and fold in the chocolate chips, peanut butter chips, flaxseed meal, coconut flaxes, and walnuts. Roll the dough into 1 ½-inch balls and arrange on the baking sheet at 2-inch intervals. Bake for 10 to 12 minutes, or until lightly golden.
Per serving: Cal 435; Net Carbs 4.6g; Fat 39g; Protein 16g

Danish Butter Cookies

Ingredients for 4 servings
¾ cup swerve confectioner's sugar
2 cups almond flour
½ cup butter, softened
1 large egg
1 tsp vanilla extract
3 oz dark chocolate
½ oz cocoa butter

Directions and Total Time: approx. 35 minutes
Preheat oven to 350 F; line a baking sheet with parchment paper. In a food processor, mix almond flour, swerve, and ¼ tsp salt. Add butter and process until resembling coarse breadcrumbs. Add eggs, vanilla, and process until smooth. Pour the batter into a piping bag and press mounds of the batter onto the baking sheets with 1-inch intervals. Bake for 10 to 12 minutes. Microwave dark chocolate and cocoa butter for 50 seconds, mixing at every 10-seconds interval. When the cookies are ready, transfer to a rack to cool and swirl the chocolate mixture.
Per serving: Cal 253; Net Carbs 0.4g; Fat 27.4g; Protein 2g

Dark Chocolate Cookies

Ingredients for 4 servings
1 ½ cups almond flour
½ cup cocoa powder
1 tsp baking soda
12 tbsp butter, softened
¾ cup swerve sugar
2 eggs
1 tsp vanilla extract
1 cup dark chocolate chips

Directions and Total Time: approx. 35 minutes
Preheat oven to 350 F; line a baking sheet with parchment paper. In a bowl, mix flour, cocoa powder, 1 tsp salt, and baking soda. In a separate bowl, cream the butter and swerve sugar until light and fluffy. Mix in the eggs, vanilla extract and then combine both mixtures. Fold in the chocolate chips until well distributed. Roll the dough into 1 ½-inch balls and arrange on the sheet at 2-inch intervals. Bake for 22 minutes until lightly golden.
Per serving: Cal 270; Net Carbs 6.7g; Fat 29g; Protein 6.2g

Ginger Cookies

Ingredients for 4 servings
4 tbsp coconut oil
2 tbsp sugar-free maple syrup
1 egg
2 tbsp water
2 ½ cups almond flour
1/3 cup swerve sugar
2 tsp ginger powder
1 tsp cinnamon powder
½ tsp nutmeg powder
1 tsp baking soda
¼ tsp salt

Directions and Total Time: approx. 25 minutes
Preheat oven to 350 F; line a baking sheet with parchment paper. In a bowl and using an electric mixer, mix coconut oil, maple syrup, egg, and water. In a separate bowl, mix flour, swerve, ginger, cinnamon, nutmeg, baking soda, and salt. Combine both mixtures until smooth. Roll the dough into 1 ½-inch balls and arrange on the sheet at 2-inch intervals. Bake for 15 minutes until lightly golden.
Per serving: Cal 141; Net Carbs 1.5g; Fat 15g; Protein 2g

Cream Cheese Cookies

Ingredients for 4 servings
¼ cup softened butter
2 oz softened cream cheese
1/3 cup xylitol
1 large egg
2 tsp vanilla extract
¼ tsp salt
1 tbsp sour cream
3 cups blanched almond flour

Directions and Total Time: approx. 25 minutes
Preheat oven to 350 F; line a baking sheet with parchment paper. In a bowl and using an electric mixer, whisk butter, cream cheese, and xylitol until fluffy and light in color. Beat in egg, vanilla, salt, and sour cream until smooth. Add flour and mix until smooth batter forms. With a cookie scoop, arrange 1 ½ tbsp of batter onto the sheet at 2-inch intervals. Bake for 15 minutes until lightly golden.
Per serving: Cal 177; Net Carbs 1.3g; Fat 17g; Protein 3g

Easy No-Bake Cookies

Ingredients for 4 servings
¾ cup coconut oil
¾ cup peanut butter
¼ cup cocoa powder
1 cup swerve brown sugar
1 tsp vanilla extract
1 ½ cup coconut flakes
2 tbsp hulled hemp seeds

Directions and Total Time: approx. 30 minutes
Preheat oven to 350 F; line two baking sheets with parchment paper. Add coconut oil and peanut butter to a pot. Melt the mixture over low heat until smoothly combined. Stir in cocoa powder, swerve sugar, and vanilla until smooth. Slightly increase the heat and simmer the mixture with occasional stirring until slowly boiling. Turn the heat off. Mix in coconut flakes and hemp seeds. Set the mixture aside to cool. Spoon the batter into silicone muffin cups and freeze for 15 minutes or until set. Serve.

Per serving: Cal 364; Net Carbs 5.5g; Fat 37g; Protein 5g

APPENDIX : RECIPES INDEX

A

All Seeds Flapjacks 103
Almond Cauliflower Cakes 14
Almond Crusted Chicken Zucchini Stacks 41
Almond Square Cookies 106
Antipasti Skewers 17
Assorted Grilled Veggies & Beef Steaks 49
Avocado & Cauliflower Salad with Prawns 66
Avocado Fries 82
Avocado Pate with Flaxseed Toasts 27
Avocado Truffles with Chocolate Coating 80

B

Bacon & Pistachio Liverwurst Truffles 91
Bacon Chicken Skillet with Bok Choy 42
Baked Chorizo with Cottage Cheese 89
Baked Creamy Brussels Sprouts 77
Baked Spicy Eggplants 92
Baked Toast Strips with Prosciutto Butter 85
Baked Tofu with Roasted Peppers 33
Barbecued Beef Pizza 48
Basil-Chili Mozzarella Bites 104
Beef & Pesto Filled Tomatoes 53
Beef Broccoli Curry 57
Beef Burgers with Roasted Brussels Sprouts 51
Beef Patties with Cherry Tomatoes 54
Beef with Broccoli Rice & Eggs 55
Beef with Parsnip Noodles 49
Bell Pepper Turkey Keto Carnitas 45
Berry Hazelnut Trifle 81
Blackberry Camembert Puffs 24
Blackberry Lemon Tarte Tatin 80
Brazilian Moqueca (Shrimp Stew) 31
Broccoli & Fish Gratin 65
Broccoli Salad with Tempeh & Cranberries 15
Broccoli Tips with Lemon Pork Chops 59
Broccoli, Spinach & Feta Salad 22
Bruschetta with Tomato & Basil 20
Buttered Greens with Almonds & Tofu Salad 18

C

Cacao Nut Bites 83
Caprese Salad with Bacon 13
Caprese Turkey Meatballs 45
Cauli Rice & Chicken Collard Wraps 40
Cauliflower & Broccoli Gratin with Seitan 76
Cauliflower Chips with Cheese Dip 97
Cauliflower Couscous & Halloumi Packets 74
Cauliflower Rice & Bacon Gratin 85
Celery Chicken Sausage Frittata 42
Chargrilled Broccoli in Tamarind Sauce 13
Charred Asparagus with Creamy Sauce 68
Cheddar and Halloumi Sticks 101
Cheese & Beef Bake 51
Cheese & Garlic Crackers 89
Cheese Quesadillas with Fruit Salad 72
Cheesy Chicken Wraps 89
Cheesy Pork Rind Bread 87
Cheesy Turkey Sausage Egg Cups 47
Chia Pudding with Blackberries 9
Chicken with Tomato and Zucchini 40
Chili Avocado with Cheese Sauce 12
Chili Avocado-Chimichurri Appetizer 99
Chili Turnip Fries 84
Chocolate Crunch Bars 105
Chocolate Walnut Biscuits 100
Chocolate, Berries & Nut Mix Bars 98
Classic Beef Ragu with Veggie Pasta 48
Classic Swedish Coconut Meatballs 50
Coconut Chocolate Fudge 82
Cowboy Cookies 107
Cranberry Coconut Parfait 83
Cream Cheese & Caramelized Onion Dip 26
Cream Cheese Cookies 109
Creamy Turkey & Broccoli Bake 47
Crispy Pancetta & Butternut Squash Roast 86

Crispy Squash Nacho Chips 99
Crunchy Rutabaga Puffs 86
Cucumber Salsa Topped Turkey Patties 44
Cumin Pork Chops 61

D

Danish Butter Cookies 108
Dark Chocolate Cookies 108

E

Easy Bacon & Cheese Balls 84
Easy No-Bake Cookies 110
Easy Rump Steak Salad 52
Egg Cauli Fried Rice with Grilled Cheese 71
Eggplant & Goat Cheese Pizza 67

F

Feta Cheese Choux Buns 29
Fish & Cauliflower Parmesan Gratin 64
Fish Fritters 66
Fried Artichoke Hearts 90

G

Garam Masala Traybake 75
Ginger Cookies 109
Goat Cheese Stuffed Peppers 90
Golden Pork Chops with Mushrooms 61
Grandma's Cauliflower Salad with Peanuts 19
Greek Salad 17
Grilled Garlic Chicken with Cauliflower 43
Gruyere Beef Burgers with Sweet Onion 58

H

Habanero Beef Cauliflower Pilaf 54
Hazelnut-Crusted Salmon 64
Heart-Shaped Red Velvet Cakes 105
Hemp Seed Zucchini Chips 103
Herbed Bolognese Sauce 50
Herby Cheesy Nuts 100
Herby Chicken Stew 32
Hot Chicken Meatball Tray 46

J

Jalapeño Nacho Wings 84
Jerk Pork Pot Roast 59

K

Keto Deviled Eggs 91

Key Lime Truffles 78

L

Lemon Muffins 10
Lemon Sponge Cake with Cream 78

M

Maple Scallion Pork Bites 60
Mascarpone and Kale Asian Casserole 74
Mashed Broccoli with Roasted Garlic 92
Mediterranean Deviled Eggs 95
Mediterranean Roasted Turnip Bites 26
Mexican Pizza 55
Mini Ricotta Cakes 25
Mint Ice Cream 67
Mixed Seed Crackers 101
Mom's Cheesy Pizza 77
Mozzarella in Prosciutto Blanket 98
Mushroom & Broccoli Pizza 73
Mushroom Broccoli Faux Risotto 95
Mushroom White Pizza 75

N

Nori Shrimp Rolls 63

O

One-Pot Spicy Brussel Sprouts with Carrots 70
Onion Rings & Kale Dip 94

P

Paleo Coconut Flour Chicken Nuggets 41
Paprika & Dill Deviled Eggs 88
Paprika Chicken & Bacon Stew 30
Paprika Roasted Nuts 94
Parmesan Green Bean Crisps 88
Parmesan Meatballs 38
Parsley Sausage Stew 31
Pepperoni Fat Head Pizza 37
Pesto Caprese Salad Stacks with Anchovies 16
Pesto Mushroom Pinwheels 102
Polish Beef Tripe 56
Pork & Pumpkin Stew with Peanuts 30
Pork Medallions with Pancetta 61
Prosciutto Appetizer with Blackberries 93
Provolone & Prosciutto Chicken Wraps 90

Pulled Pork Tenderloin with Avocado 59

R

Raspberry & Red Wine Crumble 82
Roasted Asparagus with Goat Cheese 21
Roasted Bell Pepper Salad with Olives 19
Roasted Butternut Squash with Chimichurri 35
Roasted Jalapeño & Bell Pepper Soup 15
Rosemary Cheese Chips with Guacamole 87
Rosemary Turkey Brussels Sprouts Cakes 43

S

Salmon Caesar Salad with Poached Eggs 65
Savory Gruyere & Bacon Cake 21
Savory Lime Fried Artichokes 87
Seitan Cauliflower Gratin 39
Shallot Mussel with Shirataki 63
Shitake Butter Steak 57
Simple Stuffed Eggs with Mayonnaise 86
Smoked Paprika Grilled Ribs 56
Soy Chorizo Stuffed Cabbage Rolls 97
Speedy Beef Carpaccio 20
Spicy Cheese with Tofu Balls 34
Spicy Pistachio Dip 93
Spinach Chips with Guacamole Hummus 96
Steak Carnitas 52
Sticky Maple Cinnamon Cake 106
Strawberry Blackberry Pie 81
Strawberry Faux Oats 72
Sweet & Spicy Brussel Sprout Stir-Fry 35
Sweet Onion & Goat Cheese Pizza 69
Sweet Tahini Twists 28
Swiss Pork Patties with Salad 60

T

Tangy Nutty Brussel Sprout Salad 16
Tasty Beef Cheeseburgers 53
Tasty Curried Chicken Meatballs 46
Tasty Keto Snickerdoodles 104
Tofu Eggplant Pizza 36
Tofu Jalapeño Peppers 27
Tofu Nuggets with Cilantro Dip 70
Tofu Pops 23
Tofu Radish Bowls 73
Tofu Skewers with Sesame Sauce 14
Tofu Stuffed Peppers 96
Tomato & Mozzarella Caprese Bake 68
Tomato Artichoke Pizza 36
Tuna Topped Pickles 91
Turkey with Avocado Sauce 44

V

Vegan BBQ Tofu Kabobs with Green Dip 69
Vegan Cordon Bleu Casserole 38

W

Walnut Chocolate Squares 76
Walnut Stuffed Mushrooms 39
Warm Mushroom & Yellow Pepper Salad 22
White Chocolate Chip Cookies 107
White Pizza with Mixed Mushrooms 37
Wine Shrimp Scampi Pizza 62

Y

Yellow Squash Duck Breast Stew 32
Yogurt Strawberry Pie with Basil 11

Z

Zoodle Bolognese 33
Zucchini & Dill Bowls with Goat-Feta Cheese 18
Zucchini Boats with Vegan Cheese 34
Zucchini Cake Slices 79
Zucchini Muffins 9
Zucchini-Cranberry Cake Squares 71

CPSIA information can be obtained
at www.ICGtesting.com
Printed in the USA
BVHW061610190521
607639BV00003B/645